YOUR CHILD
AND EPILEPSY

YOUR CHILD AND EPILEPSY

A Guide to Living Well

Robert J. Gumnit, M.D.

President, MINCEP® Epilepsy Care
Minneapolis, Minnesota

Clinical Professor of Neurology and Neurosurgery
University of Minnesota

demos vermande ◆

Demos Vermande, 386 Park Avenue South, New York, New York 10016

Library of Congress Cataloging-in-Publication Data

Gumnit, Robert J.
    Your child and epilepsy : a guide to living well / Robert J.
Gumnit.
        p.   cm.
    Includes bibliographical references and index.
    ISBN 0–939957–78–7 (hc). — ISBN 0–939957–76–0 (softcover)
    1. Epilepsy in children—Popular works.   I. Title.
RJ496.E6G85   1995
618.92´853—dc20   95-37697
                                                      CIP

Made in the United States of America

This book is dedicated to Frances H. Graham,
whose intelligently applied energy and strong dedication
is helping lead MINCEP® Epilepsy Care
into the twenty-first century.

CONTENTS

PREFACE

Epilepsy is not a disease, it is a constellation of symptoms. Therefore, there is no "cure" for epilepsy. Some of the causes of epilepsy can be cured. In most cases, even if a cure is not possible, complete control of seizures can be brought about. In nearly all cases, improvement in the quality of life can be obtained. Epilepsy requires long-term, continuing concerned treatment with a multi-specialty approach.

Seizures are not good for the brain and disability is not good for the soul. Major interventions are more successful when carried out early. The average patient referred to MINCEP has had seizures for fourteen years. We don't let people have gall bladder attacks for fourteen years! The modern treatment of epilepsy is as effective as our treatment of gall bladder disease.

I have adopted the practice of using male and female pronouns in alternate chapters throughout the book. His/her is an ugly construction and sentences become unnecessarily complex if one attempts to use only neuter pronouns, the third person, or the indirect voice. Seizures do not discriminate between the sexes, and neither do I.

ACKNOWLEDGMENTS

This book represents my current thinking after almost forty years in the practice of medicine, with a major focus on epilepsy for the past thirty years. I owe a debt to all of my coworkers and patients over these years who have taught me so much. When I sat down to list the names of the coworkers I wished to acknowledge, I stopped because I had a list of fifty with more to go. I began to worry that I would inadvertently overlook someone or hurt someone's feelings. You know who you are, and I hope you will understand why your name doesn't appear here.

Mr. Mike Moore provided editorial help and writing assistance. His insights were particularly helpful in Chapter 29, "Keeping Hope Alive Through Research." Florence Grey worked with me in developing and managing the research and educational aspects of the Comprehensive Epilepsy Program from 1974 until she retired almost twenty years later. MINCEP would not be what it is today, nor I the physician I am today, without her positive influences.

CHAPTER 1

YOUR CHILD CAN LIVE SUCCESSFULLY WITH EPILEPSY

To you as parents, the most important words in the title of this book are undoubtedly *child* and *epilepsy*. You want to find out more about epilepsy and what it means for your child. This book was designed to provide that information, and also to provide the motivation that will help you and your child maximize the quality of your lives.

Unless children suffer from frequent seizures that cannot be controlled (which is rare), they *can* live well with epilepsy. You can help your child to grow up believing that "there is nothing I can't do, I just need to do some things differently." To do this, you need three tools: information, the best health care possible, and a positive attitude.

I have seen these three tools used successfully by many patients and their families, and they have taught me not to focus on what is lost because of a health problem, but on what a person *has* and *can do*. Some patients, despite living with severe cases of epilepsy, lead full lives and pursue goals that are important to them. Others, with milder cases of epilepsy, experience much more disruption in their lives. The difference lies in attitude and self-image. People who choose to focus on what they can do to control epilepsy in order to enjoy their lives will see themselves not as victims, but as victors.

You can help your child achieve that kind of self-image by motivating him to focus on *can* rather than *cannot*. This book provides information to help you understand your child's epilepsy, suggestions on how to evaluate your child's health care, to find better care if necessary, and advice on helping your child to develop self-confidence and self-motivation. You are taking an important step in your family's life by reading this book. The knowledge and the ideas inspired by other patients and their families will convince you that your child *can* live well with epilepsy.

Does Your Child Have Epilepsy?

A diagnosis of epilepsy is usually made when a physician believes that a child has had two or more epileptic seizures separated in time. This was not the case in the past, when physicians tended to avoid the term *epilepsy* unless a patient had frequent seizures over an extended period. This change came about because we now realize that it does not really matter whether we call something "epilepsy" or "a seizure disorder" or something else. What matters is that we recognize that seizures have occurred and begin to consider how to respond to this reality. Today we have many effective treatments to prevent seizures or to greatly reduce their frequency, and public understanding has increased so that there is less stigma attached to the term *epilepsy*.

A *seizure* is a symptom of a temporary disturbance of brain activity. Everyone is capable of having a seizure if something occurs to disturb the brain's normal activity, such as an infection or temporary lack of oxygen. About one in eleven people will have a seizure at some time in his life. About one in twenty children will have at least one seizure, often caused by a fever.

If a child's seizure is due to an acute infection such as meningitis, future seizures may be prevented by treating the infection. If the child has a low seizure threshold in response to rising body temperature, future seizures can be prevented by providing medication and by cooling the child to prevent fever spikes during illness. Most children who experience a seizure as a result of such conditions will have only one or two seizures, and it is not correct to say that they have epilepsy. Additionally, some children have spells of breath-holding or other psychological responses that mimic seizures, but they also do not have epilepsy. The proper diagnosis of epilepsy is described in more detail in Chapter 4.

Children who continue to have seizures in response to fever or other conditions are said to have a "low seizure threshold." Some children experience seizures without any clear cause. A diagnosis of epilepsy is made if a physician determines that a child has had seizures on more than one occasion and is therefore likely to experience future seizures.

It is important to be clear about what a diagnosis of epilepsy does *not* mean. It does *not* mean that the child is "going crazy" or will be mentally retarded, nor does it mean that the child has a brain disease that cannot be controlled. Epilepsy is not contagious, and there is no reason for anyone to fear being around a person with epilepsy.

A diagnosis of epilepsy simply means that a person is more likely than others to have seizures. More than two million people (about one percent of the population) in the United States have epilepsy. When a diagnosis of epilepsy is made, it should signal the start of an aggressive effort to find the cause and to prevent future seizures.

Unfortunately, a specific cause for a child's seizures often cannot be identified. This does not mean there is no hope of preventing future seizures. Research has led to the development of a variety of medications, and it is now usually possible to find the appropriate medication or combination of medications that prevents a child from having seizures. The goal of modern epilepsy therapy is complete prevention of seizures—even one or two seizures a year is too many because of the danger of injury and the social problems that may result.

The best chance of achieving this goal for a child requires that a parent (both parents if the family is intact) and the child become closely involved as members of the health care team. Good epilepsy care is seldom as simple as being handed a prescription and giving the medication to the child at the prescribed intervals. To determine which medication to prescribe, it is usually necessary to obtain information about what the child was doing just before seizures occur, what physical symptoms are present during seizures, and how often the seizures occur. It also may be necessary to see a specialist who treats epilepsy—a neurologist or epileptologist—for tests of the child's brain activity and the function of nerves and muscles.

Even after a specific medication is prescribed, repeated visits to the physician may be necessary to determine the appropriate dosage. There are actually two goals when prescribing epilepsy medication: to prevent seizures and to allow the highest possible level of normal functioning. Epilepsy medications raise the seizure threshold by depressing certain types of brain activity. Too much can prevent the child from participating as fully as possible in school and other activities. Depending on what the parents and child report about the effects of a medication, the physician may adjust the dose, switch to a different medication, or prescribe a combination of two medications.

The process of diagnosing and treating epilepsy in children of various ages is described in more detail later in the book. What is important to understand now is that *you* must play a major role in helping to control your child's epilepsy. Your role on the health care team will be to provide accurate information about the child's seizures and other activities, to carry out the physician's instructions as closely as possible, and to learn about epilepsy so you can participate effectively in decisions about your child's health care. Chapter 7 provides more information about how to participate fully as part of the health care team.

We encourage our patients and their family members to communicate openly and assertively with health professionals. You are your child's chief advocate until he becomes mature enough to make health care decisions. Do not accept poor control of seizures or therapy that interferes with your child's alertness. Insist that all options be tried to achieve the best possible seizure control and awareness. Use positive messages to convey your concern or questions: "I really want to see if we can control Johnny's seizures without making him so sleepy."

If you feel that you have exhausted all resources available from your current health care team, ask for a referral to another team headed by a physician who specializes in epilepsy care. The Epilepsy Foundation of America or the National Association of Epilepsy Centers can refer you to centers in your area. See Chapters 6 and 26 for more information on finding the best possible care.

By aggressively seeking the best care for your child, you can set the tone for living well with epilepsy. Your positive approach will guide your child's response to life's challenges and the achievement of individual goals. Remember, focus on that one powerful word: *CAN*.

CHAPTER 2

YOUR CHILD
AND EPILEPSY

Attitude is a major factor in living with epilepsy. A child will learn to react to and understand the disorder by observing parents and other family members.

If a wall of silence or depression settles over the family after the diagnosis and little information is shared within the family setting, a child probably will think the worst things imaginable. If family members react with fear and panic when seizures occur and to the possibility of future seizures, the child will live in fear of them and develop a negative self-image. If children are unnecessarily sheltered from normal activities, they will grow to resent the epilepsy and will have little chance of maturing into happy, healthy adults.

On the other hand, if the family reacts positively and openly to the challenge, the child and her siblings stand a good chance of accepting the epilepsy and learning to live well in spite of it. If the seizures are treated matter of factly, and the family provides comfort and reassurance during and after a seizure (but then returns to everyday activities), the child will experience little emotional and

7

psychological harm. If parents keep epilepsy in perspective, and not only allow but also encourage the child to live as normally as possible, there is a very good chance for the child to reach her full potential in school and as an adult.

This is not to say that a parent needs to be Superman or Wonder Woman. Everyone makes mistakes in dealing with daily challenges and fortunately perfection is not required to rear healthy, happy children. What *is* important is that parents accept the child's epilepsy and firmly resolve to do whatever is necessary, to the best of their ability, to help the child live well. This is most successful when parents extend this resolve to themselves and to the child's siblings because a happy, healthy family life contributes enormously to any child's development.

How Do You Feel About Your Child's Epilepsy?

Parents may feel a wide range of emotions after learning that a child has epilepsy. It is understandable for them to worry and feel sad, helpless, guilty, and angry, especially if their child experiences setbacks or embarrassment. All parents feel these emotions as they see their children experience the physical and emotional pains of childhood. It can help to discuss these feelings with your spouse, a friend, someone you are close to, other parents of children with epilepsy, or a professional counselor. The important thing is not to allow these emotions to undermine your overall positive approach to life and your efforts to help your child to live successfully with epilepsy.

The challenge of helping a child with a chronic disorder may actually bring a family closer together. However, a family that was under stress or had poor interpersonal relationships before the diagnosis may find that epilepsy will add still more stress and may further divide it. Personal and family problems that existed before a diagnosis of epilepsy may worsen unless professional help is sought. A family counselor can be very helpful in sorting out your feelings and developing a positive approach to being a healthy individual and a good parent when these conditions exist.

Poor family relationships can undermine everything else that is done to help a child with epilepsy. If children feel unloved or are treated like a burden on the rest of the family, they are unlikely to cooperate with daily therapy. The resulting poor self-image is probably the biggest obstacle to successful living, not just with epilepsy, but simply with living. An honest, loving, supportive parent-child relationship is probably the most powerful medicine for building the positive self-image necessary to control and live successfully with epilepsy.

After the Storm: Planning for Success

Hearing the diagnosis of epilepsy stuns everyone at first, but as soon as you are able to think clearly about your child's health, you should start to formulate a plan for the future. Many people go through life letting events and experiences control them. They may have vague ideas about what they want out of life (happiness, wealth, good health), but they have not been honest and clear about how they can work toward achievable objectives. On the other hand, most successful people have a clear idea of what they want to achieve and how they are going to accomplish their goals. They have a plan that includes the steps they must take to reach short-term objectives, rewards for reaching those objectives, and long-term goals.

Take some time to think about what in life is important to you, what goals you want to attain, and what you want for your child or children. Define them as clearly as you can because they will provide the motivation for carrying out your plan.

Motivation is the internal force that moves an individual to accomplish things that build self-image and help achieve goals. Unlike negative, external forces such as nagging, threats, or bribery, motivation not only gets things done, but also creates energy rather than depleting it. Motivation helps a person overcome setbacks and stay on track to accomplish objectives and reach goals.

Both you and your child can be energized by planning together to set goals. The most obvious goal is to prevent seizures, but this is not the type of goal that provides the best motivation. Rather, doing well in school might be your child's goal. To achieve it, you and your child might decide to work together with your health care team to find the most effective antiseizure therapy, to study together for an hour each evening, and to meet with her teacher to ask for any special help that might be needed. As a reward for doing these things during the week, you might decide to go to a movie together on the weekend. As a reward for improvement on a report card, you might agree on a special outing or party to celebrate. If improvement is not made, focus instead on the good efforts that were made and discuss whether there are additional steps that can be taken to reach your goal. Other suggestions for motivating children of different ages are provided in Chapters 16–19.

Remember also to consider your *own* needs for motivation and achievement in life. Sometimes a challenge such as a child's epilepsy can cause a parent to focus on it to the exclusion of other areas of life. Therefore, it is a good idea to set goals that are unrelated to epilepsy, although obtaining good control of a child's seizures might be part of the plan for achieving a goal. For example, a parent might set a goal of finding a better job. To do this, it might be necessary to take certain training classes, and to be able to attend the night classes it might be necessary to improve a child's seizure control so she can stay with a babysitter. Again, forming a detailed plan with specific steps, objectives, rewards, and a goal can help a parent find the motivation necessary to cope with daily challenges while working toward bigger and better things.

Epilepsy, like other chronic diseases that require daily therapy and lifestyle changes, can cause a person and family to focus on what they need to do to accomplish specific goals in life. The discipline learned from following a treatment plan can carry over into other pursuits, including academics, sports, art, and work. Successes achieved as part of the health care team can teach a child to work effectively with others as part of a team or group, or within a personal relationship. In epilepsy, as in life, there will be setbacks and disappointments, but the child who grows up doing what is necessary to control epilepsy learns to overcome setbacks in order to achieve both short-term and long-term goals.

You can play a vital role in helping your child accept the challenge of living productively in the presence of epilepsy. The chapters that follow contain information, suggestions, and examples to help you play that role. Go back to them as often as necessary to find the facts and motivation you need to succeed. Together, you, your child, and the rest of your health care team can be an unbeatable force.

CHAPTER 3

UNDERSTANDING EPILEPSY

The word *epilepsy* comes from the ancient Greek word *epilepsia*, which means *seizure*. The ancient Greeks thought that a seizure was caused by a god entering the person, so epilepsy was considered a sacred disease. In medieval times, epilepsy was called the "falling sickness" and was thought to be caused by a demon entering the body. Today we know much more about the medical causes of seizures and how they can be prevented.

Many notable figures in history are thought to have had epilepsy, including Socrates, Alexander the Great, Julius Caesar, Alfred Nobel, and Thomas Edison. Likewise, many famous people today have epilepsy, including writers, artists, scientists, politicians, and athletes, as do millions of average people who are successful in their chosen careers and happy with their lives. It is important to recognize their achievements because they can help us understand that seizures can be controlled and that individuals who have them can lead full and productive lives.

Parents understandably experience many emotions and have many questions when a child is first diagnosed with epilepsy. They may feel guilty and ask if there is something they could have done to prevent the disorder. Except in cases where the child's epilepsy was caused by a problem such as a head injury that could have been prevented by a bicycle helmet or seat belt or by an infection that could have been prevented by proper immunization, there is seldom anything that could have prevented the onset of epilepsy.

Parents often ask if a child will outgrow epilepsy or if the disorder can be cured. This is rarely the case, although some children who experience absence seizures (in which they lose awareness for brief periods) may outgrow them. Most people with epilepsy can be treated effectively with medications that prevent seizures while allowing a normal lifestyle, and some cases of epilepsy can be cured, or at least made less severe, through surgery.

Sometimes there are no clear explanations, only educated guesses, as to why a child experiences seizures. Also, it may take some time to learn enough about a child's epilepsy to treat it effectively. In any case, the best way to help a child with epilepsy is to ask questions and gather information on how to control the disorder. This chapter will get you started in that direction.

What Is a Seizure?

Surprisingly, few people ask what a seizure actually *is*. Parents who have witnessed their child having a seizure are usually more concerned about the behavior during the seizure than by the internal disorder that causes it. A better understanding of seizures and the different types of epilepsy will help you become actively involved in managing your child's epilepsy.

Seizures can be divided into two general categories: epileptic and nonepileptic. An *epileptic seizure* is a sudden episode of disturbed brain activity that results in abnormal behavior, and in which the main problem lies within the child's brain. A *nonepileptic seizure* is an episode of abnormal behavior that is not caused by a disturbance in brain activity, but by some other problem. For example, nonepileptic seizures can be caused by an abrupt drop in blood pressure, an imbalance of body fluids or chemicals, or certain psychological responses.

Several tests can be done to determine whether a child has epileptic or nonepileptic seizures (some people have both). These include blood and urine tests, neurologic examinations that show how a child's brain controls muscle and nerve responses, and especially an EEG (electroencephalogram) analysis of brain activity. Various types of X-ray studies and scans that produce pictures of the brain and show how it is working are also helpful. These tests are described in detail in Chapter 5.

Epileptic seizures are caused by sudden, uncontrolled bursts of electrical activity from brain cells. Because the brain controls all behavior, an epileptic seizure causes a person to behave in an unusual way. Some people can feel a seizure coming on through a sensation called an *aura*. This sensation is actually the beginning of the seizure caused by abnormal activity in one part of the brain. The warning is usually the same every time an individual has a seizure, but each person experiences a different aura, or none at all. For some people, the aura is all there is to the seizure, while others have a seizure with no warning. Your child may be able to communicate this feeling when it occurs. Encourage him to do so because it can help you and others to prevent injury during a seizure.

A seizure may cause many different behavioral changes. The child may be unable to focus attention and may stare blankly, not responding to other people. Or the child may lose control of muscles or the bladder. Muscle spasms may occur or the child may have convulsions in which all or part of the body shakes rhythmically but uncontrollably. Many people lose consciousness during a seizure.

Most seizures are brief and last less than a minute. When the seizure is over and the child regains awareness or consciousness, he may cry and be panicky and confused, have difficulty speaking, have a headache, experience weakness in some part of the body, and may be very tired. Most people do not remember what happened to them just before and during a seizure.

Is Epilepsy a Disease?

Epilepsy should not really be described as a "disease" because recurrent seizures can be caused by many very different conditions.

The term *epilepsy* refers to a chronic (lasting a long time) disorder in which the individual either has recurrent seizures caused by disturbances in brain activity or would have such seizures if not controlled by medications.

We would not say that a person had epilepsy if, for example, two seizures occurred during an illness such as meningitis, but stopped after the illness was treated. We *would* make the diagnosis of epilepsy if a person had two seizures weeks or months apart. In other words, a seizure is a *symptom* of a problem that is causing a disturbance in the brain. If physicians cannot find a short-term cause for the seizure and the person has more, physicians would say that the patient has the disorder called epilepsy. A more complete description of the disorder would include the type of epilepsy and the kind of seizures the child experiences.

When a child first has a seizure, it is very important to see a physician to try to determine what caused the seizure. He will take a complete history of the child's health and the health of family members. Parents or others who witnessed the seizure should provide as complete a description of the seizure as possible to help the physician make a diagnosis. Treatment depends, of course, on whether the physician determines that the child has had an epileptic or nonepileptic seizure.

Epilepsy Syndromes

Physicians categorize patients as having different epilepsy *syndromes* in order to help determine treatment and predict outcome. Syndromes are defined by the type of seizures (partial, generalized, unknown) and factors such as age of onset, family history, laboratory findings, and EEG results.

What Are the Different Kinds of Seizures?

Seizures are described or classified by the behavioral and EEG changes that occur during the seizure. The following descriptions are simplified from the seizure classifications established by physicians who specialize in treating epilepsy.

1. *Partial seizures* begin in one part of the brain. They can be classified as simple partial, complex partial, or secondarily generalized tonic-clonic. *Simple partial seizures* cause a single kind of movement or a strange sensation such as emotion, smell, taste, or dizziness; the patient does not lose consciousness. In *complex partial seizures*, the person loses awareness as the seizure begins or loses awareness during a partial seizure. Almost two-thirds of people with epilepsy have complex partial seizures. Partial seizures that secondarily generalize proceed to what are called *tonic-clonic convulsions* that cause the body to become rigid (tonic), usually causing the person to fall to the ground and then to begin shaking or jerking as the muscles relax rhythmically (clonic).

2. *Generalized seizures* affect the whole body at the onset and cause an immediate loss of consciousness. They are characterized by impaired consciousness and affect the whole body. The person may have an *absence seizure*, in which awareness of surroundings is cut off; jerking of whole muscle groups (*clonic seizures*); muscle rigidity (*tonic seizure*); a generalized *tonic-clonic seizure*, in which the body becomes stiff (tonic phase) and he falls, followed by alternating stiffening and relaxation (clonic phase); or an *atonic* seizure, in which all the muscles suddenly relax, causing a collapse and fall.

3. *Unclassified seizure* is the last category, so named because not enough information is available about the person's seizures to classify them.

A person with epilepsy may experience only one kind of seizure or several different kinds, either during the same episode or at different times. Every effort must be made by the physician, family, and person with epilepsy to determine what kinds of seizures occur in order to achieve the best treatment for the seizures.

Helping Your Child to Cope with Epilepsy

Epileptic seizures can be both dangerous and embarrassing because they involve loss of control. The child may feel embarrassed, ashamed, or angry, especially if other children or unthinking adults add to the problem by ridiculing him or making a fuss about the seizure. Public education is helping people to understand epilepsy, and you and your child can play a big part in teaching people about seizures.

First, make sure that you, the rest of your family, and anyone who cares for your child know the simple first-aid steps to be taken when a seizure occurs (see Chapter 11). Second, talk to your child about the seizures, and make sure that he understands that they are not his fault and that they are not some kind of punishment. Depending on the child's age, teach him how to tell people about a seizure that has occurred. Talking openly and honestly about epilepsy and seizures—and how other people react to them—will help your child adjust and overcome any shame or fear.

As you and your child begin to understand and accept epilepsy, you will become better able to handle situations as they arise. You will also become better able to help as part of the health care team, and your child can become involved more as he matures. Treatment for seizures should ordinarily begin as soon as a diagnosis is made. Again, the goal of treatment is to control seizures completely without preventing awareness and learning. The next chapter describes what is known about the causes of epilepsy and how the disorder is diagnosed.

CHAPTER 4

THE CAUSES AND DIAGNOSIS OF EPILEPSY

One of the first challenges for your health care team will be to try to determine what has caused your child's seizures. There are many possible causes of seizures, but in about half the cases no specific cause can be positively identified. If a cause can be found, that information can be helpful in determining treatment.

This chapter discusses what is known about the causes of epilepsy and describes the procedures and tests that can be used to diagnose it and to identify kinds of seizures.

What Causes Epilepsy?

The known causes of epilepsy include:

1. Inherited diseases such as phenylketonuria (PKU), tuberous sclerosis, and neurofibromatosis can cause a person to have recurrent seizures.

2. An inherited tendency to develop epilepsy. About 2 percent of the general population develops epilepsy by age forty. When one parent or a brother or sister has epilepsy, there is about a 5 percent chance that a child will also develop epilepsy by having inherited a lower than normal seizure threshold. This inherited tendency is more likely to cause epilepsy to develop in childhood than later in life. You may wish to consult a genetic counselor for more specific information about your family's situation.

3. Problems occurring during fetal development. Most of these occur for unknown reasons, although a few may be caused by the mother's being exposed to toxic substances such as street drugs and alcohol, or by infections or injury.

4. Problems occurring during birth, such as lack of oxygen, damage from forceps delivery, or other injury to the baby's brain.

5. Head injuries at any time of life that are severe enough to cause an injury to the brain. A seizure may occur at the time of a head injury or even two or three years later, but the person does not have epilepsy unless repeated seizures occur at different times.

6. A tumor (abnormal growth of tissue) in the brain.

7. A blood clot or abnormal blood vessel formation in the brain.

Treat the Cause or Treat the Seizures?

Specific causes such as a brain tumor or blood clot can often be treated directly, in which case treating the *cause* of the epilepsy may prevent further seizures.

When epilepsy has a more general cause, such as an inherited tendency to have seizures or generalized brain damage that causes repeated seizures, the strategy is to find a treatment that will prevent the seizures. This same strategy also applies if no specific cause can be identified. If your physician has identified the cause of your child's epilepsy, accept that information as a positive step toward finding the best possible treatment.

Even if the epilepsy could not have been prevented, a professional counselor or social worker can be helpful if emotional or social problems are standing in the way of controlling your child's epilepsy. It is important to resolve these problems so that nothing stands in the way of helping your child. Developing a positive attitude is crucial for you, your child, and any other members of the family to proceed in a healthy manner.

Resolving to find the best possible care for your child and to help her live the best possible life is one effective way of overcoming an accident. Some people find that it also helps to make a special effort to educate others about preventing similar accidents or disabilities.

The Importance of Complete and Accurate Diagnosis

Whether or not a specific or general cause of your child's epilepsy can be identified, it is important to know as much as possible about seizures. Diagnosis involves much more than the conclusion that someone has epilepsy. In order to decide on the appropriate treatment to control your child's seizures, the kind or kinds of seizures must first be determined.

The diagnosis of epilepsy is sometimes very clear because there is a good description of the child's seizure. If proper treatment is prescribed and no more seizures occur, there may be no need for extensive diagnostic tests. If the diagnosis is not clear and the initial treatment does not prevent further seizures, further diagnostic tests will be necessary. These tests may even determine that your child does *not* have epilepsy.

Why Are They Asking All These Questions?

When a child first has a seizure, it is likely to be a very distressing time for the family. If the seizure is severe, causing convulsions or unconsciousness, the child should be taken to a hospital emergency room. A seizure usually lasts a little more than a minute, and the child and family might not be able to describe it very well. However, any description of your child's behavior or any feelings described before, during, and after the seizure is very helpful.

If the seizure was severe, your child will probably be admitted for observation and diagnostic tests. If it was not severe enough to bring your child to the hospital, a diagnosis may be attempted in a physician's office, or the physician may decide to hospitalize the child for further care and diagnostic tests. Antiepileptic drug therapy may begin at once to avoid the potential danger of further seizures.

The first part of the diagnostic process is to obtain a complete medical history of both the child and the family. Because epilepsy sometimes runs in families, it is important to provide as much information about the family as possible. The physician or nurse may ask questions about your child's behavior, problems with bed-wetting, history of head injury, health problems as an infant, family health problems, mental health, and the mother's use of alcohol, street drugs, or medications.

The questions may not always seem related to epilepsy, but the answers can help a physician familiar with the disorder to make a clear diagnosis. Withholding information out of fear or embarrassment may hinder efforts to prevent seizures.

After the medical history has been obtained, the physician will perform a complete physical examination that emphasizes the nervous system. Several tests can be done to evaluate the condition of the nerves leading from the brain to different parts of the body.

What Can Blood and Urine Tests Tell About a Seizure?

Whether your child is seen in the hospital or in a physician's office, laboratory tests will be ordered to detect any problems that may have contributed to the seizure. These may include infection, organ failure, mineral imbalance, high or low blood sugar, or any other of a large number of abnormalities that can be detected by analysis of the blood or urine.

When Should More Diagnostic Tests Be Pursued?

Further diagnostic tests should be done if a diagnosis of epilepsy has been made and drug therapy begun but your child's seizures are not under control after three months (or sooner if the seizures are occurring at least once every week or two). If a neurologist was not involved in the initial diagnosis, this is definitely a time to find one, preferably one who specializes in epilepsy.

The neurologist may repeat many of the diagnostic tests done earlier. This is especially true with children because they are more difficult to diagnose. The neurologist will try to clarify the seizure type to see if the appropriate medication is being used.

If antiepileptic medications do not control your child's seizures within nine months, she should be seen at a comprehensive epilepsy center by a neurologist who specializes in treating epilepsy (an epileptologist). Specialized diagnostic tests will be done to reevaluate the diagnosis. These tests will determine whether your child is one of a minority of people who have epileptic seizures that are especially difficult to control.

Why Is Diagnosis Sometimes So Complicated?

Epilepsy is a complex disorder that often includes more than one type of seizure. To treat all your child's seizures properly, your physician must find out which parts of the brain are affected and what type of seizure or seizures your child has. Only then will it be possible to develop a treatment strategy to provide maximum seizure control. The next chapter describes the range of treatment options available for epilepsy today. Chapter 8 describes special tests in more detail.

CHAPTER 5

THE HOLISTIC APPROACH TO EPILEPSY TREATMENT

The treatment of chronic disorders today is much different than it was thirty years ago. Most physicians then would have said that the treatment for diabetes was to take insulin, and the treatment for epilepsy was to take antiseizure medication. Over the years it has become clear that even when people take the appropriate medication, their lives are not always ideal. People with a wide variety of chronic disorders have helped health professionals understand that nearly all areas of patients' and families' lives are affected by the presence of disease. Therefore, effective treatment now addresses all areas of the individual's and family's health and lifestyle.

How Can You Treat an Individual's Lifestyle?

Treating all parts of a person's lifestyle is called *holistic medicine*. The word *holistic* refers to an emphasis on how the function of the parts relate to the function of the whole. In medicine, this means that it is important to consider how a disease or disorder affects all parts of the body and all parts of the individual's healthy lifestyle.

For children, the single most important factor defining their lifestyle is, of course, their family. A child's relationships with parents, siblings, and other relatives define much of what the child does and how the child feels about himself. Other factors include how the child interacts with other children and adults, how healthy the child is in general, and how he has developed physically, intellectually, and emotionally. Therefore, when a child is diagnosed with epilepsy, it is important to learn more about the child and his lifestyle. Then the health care team, including the child and family members, can prepare the best treatment plan to reach the goal of a healthy, happy life. The treatment plan might include taking one or more medications, following a healthy diet, meeting with a child and/or family counselor, and enjoying regular opportunities for exercise and social interaction. The goals of such a holistic treatment plan are:

1. To prevent seizures or reduce their frequency and severity as much as possible;

2. To maximize the child's alertness and ability to learn in order to mature normally in all areas;

3. To help the child and family eat the right foods and develop good living habits in order to be as healthy as possible;

4. To help the child and family members adjust to living with epilepsy and learn how to provide the support each person needs from other family members; and,

5. To continually evaluate and try to improve, if necessary, in all of these areas, so that the child with epilepsy and the family can live well.

When Should Medications Be Started?

Antiseizure medications should be prescribed as soon as the physician concludes that a child is at risk of having further seizures.

In other words, antiseizure therapy should be started if the child has had more than one seizure at different times and there is no acute illness or other apparent cause. This is very important because the medication often prevents further seizures, preventing the child from being exposed to their possible physical and emotional consequences.

In addition to prescribing medication early, it is important that the effectiveness of the medication be evaluated often and changes made if necessary. The different types of medications available to treat epilepsy and the choices and decisions that go into an effective medication plan are described in Chapter 9. In general, however, the two most important questions to ask in evaluating a child's medication are:

1. Is the child continuing to have seizures while taking the medication as prescribed?

2. Is the medication preventing the child from participating in normal physical and mental activities?

If the answer to either or both of the above is yes, and enough time has passed to properly evaluate the medication, discuss the situation with your child's physician. Many options are available, and it is not necessary to settle for continuing seizures or reduced function unless and until all options have been tried. Chapter 9 describes these options, which include changing the dose, changing the medication, combining medications, use of a special diet, and surgical treatment.

How does good general health improve epilepsy care? Everyone has more energy and enthusiasm for life when they are healthy and physically fit. Children with epilepsy and their family members benefit in the same way. If a mother, father, or sibling gets sick often or does not have much energy, it can be difficult for them to help a child with epilepsy. But if they are fit and feel good about life, they can be a positive influence on the child.

Likewise, if a child with epilepsy often catches colds and other minor illnesses, he will not have much energy to devote to school and to playing with other children. Also, the need to take prescribed or over-the-counter medications can interfere with antiseizure medications. This can be managed occasionally, but it can become difficult if the child needs to take other medications often.

Eating nutritious foods and getting plenty of exercise and sleep give a child the energy to enjoy life. These healthy habits, along with good hygiene, can also help prevent minor illnesses. If a child is in good general health, it is much easier to deal with any problems related to epilepsy. This is why we believe so strongly in holistic care.

If you think your family's nutritional habits could be improved, ask your physician for advice and possibly a referral to a dietitian. If you are concerned about what type of activities you or your child can do to get exercise, ask your physician's advice. If your family seems to catch every "bug" that comes along, perhaps your nurse, physician, or dietitian can evaluate your general health and provide some advice. If your family members always seem to be arguing with each other or are sad, withdrawn, or angry about life, perhaps a counselor can help you develop healthier ways to deal with life's challenges. Each member of your family can become part of the health care team that *prevents* health problems as well as *treats* those that occur. Prevention is much easier and cheaper than treatment. When epilepsy is part of your life, prevention of seizures and other health problems is even more important.

Strive for the best, most comprehensive health care possible. The next chapter provides some suggestions for finding your way to high quality, holistic health care.

CHAPTER 6

FINDING YOUR WAY
TO HIGH QUALITY CARE

Unlike in the past, today there are many effective treatments for epilepsy. There is also a more positive attitude about caring for people with epilepsy. Many physicians who treat chronic disease now understand the importance of a team approach to providing high quality care. We have learned that positive results come when a family and a child with epilepsy become involved in a team effort to achieve a healthy and happy life.

Your challenge is to gain access to the kind of competent and comprehensive care your child needs. To do so, you need to know how the health care system works and must be willing to assert yourself to obtain high quality care. Unfortunately, some families find it difficult to get adequate health care, especially if they do not have health insurance. Even those who have insurance need to know how to use it to their best advantage.

To succeed in the search for high quality care, you must be willing to hunt for it—and fight for it, if necessary. This chapter provides information and tips to help you succeed.

Coping in Our Rapidly Changing Health Care System

The United States health care system in undergoing many changes. Increasing costs have strained the resources of government programs and have made health insurance an important concern of individuals and families. For people whose employer does not provide adequate coverage or who are unemployed, a major health problem can cause financial catastrophe. Until basic changes are made in our health care system, some people will continue to be denied basic health care.

Families affected by chronic disorders such as epilepsy often are either denied health insurance or asked to pay such high rates that the insurance is as unaffordable as the care it is intended to cover. Increasing costs and the social inequities they have caused have led to a national debate on health care in the United States. It is hoped that high quality health care will someday be provided to everyone. Until that happens, you owe it to yourself and to your child to fight for the best care you can get right now.

Those who understand our current health care system are in the best position to get the most benefit from it. It is important to realize that health care is a *business*. Like other businesses, health care professionals have organized themselves into groups that share the costs of providing care. Physicians today tend to work with a small group of partners or to be affiliated with a clinic or large health care center. Like other businesses, these groups compete to provide services to the public.

Competition in health care is seen in two major ways. First, groups of health professionals compete to provide services to patients covered by insurance programs offered by employers or through government programs. These programs are increasingly organized as managed care plans, which compete to provide services for the lowest fixed annual payments. The family needs to study the quality of care they offer, especially asking about access to specialists and specialized centers.

The second type of competition takes place among individual physicians to see who can best meet a patient's health care needs.

We will discuss this in some detail because by knowing how to take advantage of this competition you can increase your chances of getting quality health care.

Types of Health Care Insurance or Service Plans

Traditional Health Insurance (Indemnity Plans)

A few companies still provide the traditional type of health insurance called an "indemnity plan." These plans pay most or all of an employee's and family members' medical expenses and allow them to see any physician they choose. Indemnity insurance provides the greatest flexibility, but it is usually the most expensive type of plan.

Managed Care Providers

Because of the rapidly rising costs of indemnity plans, many companies and government programs are signing contracts with managed health care service companies; the differences among them are explained in Chapter 22. These groups are generally called health maintenance organizations (HMOs) or preferred provider organizations (PPOs).

An HMO or PPO sells health services to employers or to the government, which in turn provide free or reduced cost memberships to their employers or to citizens who qualify for a specific government program. Members are then entitled to go to those (generally limited) physicians, clinics, and hospitals that have signed contracts with the managed care plan. The plan pays only part of the costs—and sometimes none of them—if a member goes to a physician who does not have a contract with the HMO or PPO. The plan also pays only part or none of the costs for certain services that are not covered under the member's contract. Some contracts are quite restrictive and limit access to specialized care. Many HMOs or PPOs require members to first see a family practitioner, and only if that physician decides that the patient needs to see a specialist does the plan pay for specialized care.

It is important to understand that these plans *do not all have the same rules and restrictions* and that one managed care company often negotiates for different levels and types of services with a specific employer or government program. If you are given a choice among several plans, it is crucial to shop for the best one for you and your family. Unfortunately, most of these plans describe their benefits in vague and generally reassuring terms. Learn to look beneath the surface. Ask tough questions of your Human Resources Department.

If you are unemployed or your employer does not provide health insurance, check with your local county welfare office to find out if you or your family members qualify for any government programs. The federal and state governments provide medical services to people with low incomes through medical assistance programs. Many states have established medical programs for children, especially for those with chronic health disorders. Some states offer insurance to people who have been refused coverage by commercial insurance companies. You need to find out what services your family is eligible for and how to use them.

If you become a member of an HMO, you need to learn the rules and restrictions for services. If you do not follow the rules (such as when and where to go for emergency and urgent care), you may be required to pay large bills for those services. It is also important to learn about and use the services that are provided under your HMO contract. A few HMOs stress preventive health services, such as health and nutrition education classes, regular checkups and immunizations, smoking cessation programs, and sometimes drug and alcohol treatment programs and mental health counseling. A few offer special programs for people with chronic disorders such as diabetes, arthritis, and epilepsy. These services and programs can play a major role in helping you solve problems that are preventing you and your family from living well with epilepsy.

Of course, in searching for and choosing an insurance policy or managed care plan from among those offered by your employer or government program, you should focus on those that provide the best services for children with epilepsy. If you are switching coverage or looking for a new job, inquire about coverage for preexisting conditions such as epilepsy. Find out if prescription medications are covered, especially for brand-name versus generic forms of anti-seizure medications (this is discussed further in Chapter 9). Also ask about the type of physicians and other health professionals your child will be able to visit. Can you go "out of plan" to a comprehensive epilepsy center?

How Do Health Professionals Compete for Patients?

In the past, most people went to one physician for all of their medical problems and for most of their lives, seeing another physician only if they went to the hospital or moved. Today physicians called generalists, family physicians, or primary care physicians still see patients for checkups, to diagnose problems, and to care for limited disorders. But there are also many physicians who specialize in treating specific medical problems. A very few specialize in treating epilepsy.

No one kind of physician is best for all problems. A child with epilepsy needs two types of health care: (1) overall care to prevent and treat general medical problems, and (2) specialized care for epilepsy.

There is great value in having one generalist or family physician who supervises health care for you and your family. She can direct you through the health care system and refer you to specialists when necessary. This can be especially helpful for a child with epilepsy. It can be worthwhile to ask to see several different family physicians until you find one with whom you and your child are comfortable, and who is the most helpful in providing services and information and referring you to specialists when necessary.

General physicians who are more specialized include pediatricians, who see children under the age of eighteen; internists, who diagnose and treat medical problems in adults but do not perform surgery; and gerontologists, who primarily see patients over age sixty-five. Generalists diagnose and treat a wide variety of illnesses but are expected to refer patients to specialists for more extensive diagnosis, treatment, and advice about more serious problems.

You may request a referral to a pediatrician, for example, if you do not feel that your family physician is providing the best possible care and information about your child's growth and development. When a child requires diagnosis or treatment for a serious or less common problem such as epilepsy, you should request referral to a physician who specializes in the disorder.

You will probably be referred to a neurologist, a physician who treats diseases of the brain and other parts of the nervous system such as epilepsy, stroke, Alzheimer's disease, Parkinson's disease, and multiple sclerosis (MS), as well as many other diseases and disorders. To qualify as a neurologist, a physician must have at least four years of special training after medical school and must pass an examination given by the American Board of Psychiatry and Neurology. Pediatric neurologists specialize in treating children.

Other neurologists concentrate on helping only patients with epilepsy. These "epileptologists" belong to professional epilepsy associations such as the American Epilepsy Society, and they usually work closely with the Epilepsy Foundation of America (EFA) and its local affiliate. They are often best able to treat patients with epilepsy. There are approximately 650,000 physicians in the United States in 1995; only 10,000 are neurologists and fewer than 500 are epileptologists. Epileptologists can be found in most major cities.

Making the Choice

Many factors can affect your choice of a physician, including where you live, if you are a member of an HMO, and whether your family has other specialized needs in addition to epilepsy.

For regular medical care, you should establish a relationship with a physician or clinic near your home. If you live in a rural area, you may have few choices, but your physician should still be able to consult with a neurologist about your child's epilepsy treatment. It may also be helpful to travel to a specialized epilepsy center for regular evaluations of your child's epilepsy control.

If you live in a city, you usually have many physicians from which to choose, especially if you have indemnity (traditional) health insurance or if you pay for the care yourself. Ask your friends and neighbors to recommend a family physician, and if you know someone else who has a child with epilepsy, ask them which physician they see. Remember that if you or your child feel uncomfortable or unhappy with a physician, you are free to search for another.

Even within the restrictions of an HMO or other health insurance coverage, you should be able to choose physicians who are right for you. Be assertive in finding out about your rights and which physicians are available to you. Then take time to get to know them and give them a chance to provide the best care for you and your family members. Be especially assertive and careful about finding the best care for your child with epilepsy.

Many people with epilepsy receive excellent routine health care and epilepsy monitoring from general practice physicians, but it is important that they be able to see a specialist if necessary. This is especially important for a child who has recently been diagnosed with epilepsy. Making a thorough and proper diagnosis, prescribing and adjusting medications, and evaluating epilepsy control require training, experience, and specialized equipment. An epileptologist can get you and your child started on the right track and then work with a general practitioner to make sure they stay that way.

If you are not satisfied with your access to specialized care or if you are not sure if your child's physician is communicating with a neurologist, ask your physician about her knowledge of epilepsy. Find out how much training in epilepsy care she has, how she keeps up with current epilepsy information, and if she consults with other physicians when making decisions about your child's care. These questions should be asked not as challenges to your physician's ability but as sincere signs that you want to make sure your child is getting the best possible epilepsy treatment.

If your insurance plan limits your access to specialized care, express your dissatisfaction to plan representatives and especially to your employer. Start with your physician, but realize that she probably has little control over the type of coverage you have. Pursue your questions with your employer and with representatives of your health insurance company. Go as far up the chain of authority as you must to gain satisfaction. You may receive assistance from the state health department or other agencies, or from the insurance commissioner who supervises HMOs. An especially effective argument is that your child's epilepsy needs could be met less expensively if her control were improved by seeing a specialist. Don't take no for an answer if you are convinced that you have a reasonable request for quality health care.

Finding Epilepsy Resources

The Epilepsy Foundation of America (EFA) is a good source of information about neurologists and epileptologists in your area. If possible, attend local EFA meetings and volunteer your help. This is a great way to find out about health professionals who specialize in epilepsy care, to get information and advice about your child, and to learn about advances and research in epilepsy. (See Chapter 24 for more information about the EFA.) You can call the National Association of Epilepsy Centers (612-525-4526) for a list of specialized centers.

Many neurologists provide good epilepsy care. However, neurologists provide care in several different settings, which may affect the quality of care your child receives. Some neurologists work alone, seeing patients in a private office. Others work in a larger office with other neurologists and possibly nurse-clinicians, who can provide education and spend additional time discussing your child's health problems.

Special epilepsy centers have been established in some cities. These centers bring together epileptologists, nurse-clinicians, nurse-educators, psychologists, pharmacists, laboratory technicians, and other professionals, who work with patients and family members as a team to provide the comprehensive services often needed for optimal epilepsy care. Some have a national reputation, which you could find out about from the EFA or the NAEC.

An epilepsy center is likely to have the most experience in managing difficult cases. Epilepsy centers are often affiliated with a large medical center, where extensive diagnostic procedures can be done, and where more complex medication combinations can be monitored and surgical treatment considered. They are also usually involved in research, including clinical trials of new drugs that may improve epilepsy control. If you find such an epilepsy center, ask if it is a member of the National Association of Epilepsy Centers and if it meets the association's guidelines.

Each of the settings described here has good and bad points, and you need to find the one that works best for your child. Factors to consider in making a choice are:

✧ Length of time needed to get an appointment;

✧ Telephone access to nurse-clinician or neurologist for help, especially in an emergency;

✧ Willingness of neurologist to work with your child's regular physician to monitor epilepsy control;

✧ Feeling that your child's individual needs and preferences are considered and that you and your child are part of the team working together to control epilepsy;

✧ Satisfaction that your child's epilepsy needs are met and your questions are answered at each visit;

✧ Availability of laboratory services for evaluation of your child's treatment;

✧ Ability to provide for other needs related to epilepsy, such as education, psychological and social counseling, financial assistance or advice, and help in working within the requirements of your health insurance plan;

✧ Knowledge and effectiveness of the physician treating your child.

Don't Settle for So-So Care

Never stop evaluating your satisfaction with your child's general health care and epilepsy control. Be prepared to pay for special services that your family needs but for which your insurance company or managed care plan refuses to pay. There is nearly always something that can be done differently, either by you or by your physician. The next chapter provides advice on making the most of your relationships with the people helping you and your child live well with epilepsy.

CHAPTER 7

BEING AN EFFECTIVE MEMBER OF YOUR CHILD'S HEALTH CARE TEAM

Many parents take a passive approach to dealing with physicians and nurses. They take their child to the physician, sit quietly during the examination, answer any questions they are asked, and leave with a prescription for medication or "orders" from the physician. They act this way because that is how they have learned to act in the past—they think they are being good patient-parents. Unfortunately, a parent who takes this approach is actually withholding the participation of the two most important members of the epilepsy health care team: not the physician and nurse, but the child and parent.

How You and Your Child Can Join Your Epilepsy Health Care Team

Make an effort to become an effective member of the team taking care of your child's epilepsy, since the team's success depends to a great extent on the information you provide and the actions you take. You know your child best. You can report his feelings, behaviors, problems, and triumphs. Until your child is old enough to convey this information, you are the spokesperson and advocate.

Proper diagnosis and treatment of epilepsy depend on accurate reporting of seizures, any side effects from medications, and general health problems. This information enables the rest of the team to develop a plan that best meets the needs of your child. By expressing your concerns about your child—whether or not they seem to be related to epilepsy—you can help the team improve your child's plan so that he can live well with epilepsy.

Think for a moment about how you feel about your child's health care team. Ask yourself the following questions about the health professionals you and your child are seeing:

✧ Do you feel comfortable talking with your physician and nurses?

✧ Does your child seem comfortable, or at least not excessively fearful, around the team members? Do they make an effort to help your child overcome fears and feel safe and involved rather than just an object to be poked and prodded?

✧ Do you feel comfortable with their professional knowledge in treating epilepsy and in their willingness and ability to refer you to others for specialized care?

✧ Have they provided you with understandable, useful educational information about epilepsy? Have they talked to you about how to explain epilepsy to your child?

✧ Do they involve you in decision-making and planning, or do they just give instructions without asking how you feel about the arrangements being made?

✧ Do they ask about aspects of your child's life that are not directly related to epilepsy, such as social involvement, learning abilities, behavior at home and in public?

✧ Do they take time to answer your questions? Do they talk to you in terms you can understand?

✧ Can you reach your child's nurse or physician to ask questions and report problems?

✧ Are you satisfied with your child's epilepsy control?

Next, ask these questions about yourself:

✧ Do you understand all the services your child's health care team can provide? Do you know whom to contact for what?

✧ Are you on time for appointments?

✧ Do you prepare for visits by keeping good records and writing down the questions you want to ask?

✧ Are you honest and complete when presenting information about your child and discussing problems?

✧ Do you take the time to learn about epilepsy through educational materials?

✧ Do you occasionally take someone with you (your spouse, the child's brother or sister, another relative or friend who cares for your child, or your child's day-care provider or teacher) if you need help describing seizures or figuring out how to solve problems your child is having?

✧ Do you listen carefully to instructions and write down information you might forget? Do you encourage your child (if old enough) to write down and ask questions or make suggestions?

✧ Do you help your child to take medications on time and to follow other parts of the health plan?

✧ Do you ask for help for your child, yourself, or your family when needed for medical, emotional, social, or financial reasons?

✦ Are you happy with your child's epilepsy control? Is your child happy with his or her epilepsy control?

The last question in both lists is the key question in evaluating your child's team. Think about it occasionally, and answer truthfully. There is no need for change if you are truly satisfied that everything possible has been done to maximize your child's epilepsy control and general health and development.

If you are like most parents, however, there are several areas in which your child's health care team could be improved. Here are some suggestions for improving your relationship with each team member.

Is Your Relationship with Your Child's Physician Satisfactory?

Probably the most common complaints parents have is that their child's physician does not spend enough time with them and does not listen carefully to their questions or concerns. If you feel this way, do not assume that your child's physician is uncaring. There may be several reasons for a visit that feels rushed, and there are several things you can do to make better use of your time and that of your child's physician.

First, keep in mind that if your child is feeling fine and has no problems with epilepsy control, there is no need for your physician to spend much time with you. A quick exam and some encouraging words for your child and you—"Keep up the good work!"—are all you need.

If you do have questions to ask or problems to discuss, plan your child's visit carefully. When you make an appointment, explain why you are bringing your child. Schedule visits well in advance if possible. A busy clinic may not be able to schedule you for a routine visit for two weeks or a month, but in a crisis you should always be able to see a physician or nurse-clinician or be referred elsewhere to have the problem dealt with.

A first visit usually requires more than an hour. Not all this time will be with the physician. You and your child may also see a nurse-clinician, have blood drawn, and look at some educational materials. Make the most of this first visit by making sure to have your child's complete medical records transferred; or, better yet, pick them up and take them with you. Arrive early enough to allow time to fill out new patient forms and medical history questionnaires. Be sure to tell the nurse and physician if you have a hearing or vision problem, do not read well, do not understand English well, or if you and/or your child have any other problem that might interfere with your participation on the health care team. There is always something that can be done to increase your participation.

If you have financial questions about your child's care, ask to see the business manager or other appropriate person. Most clinics will help you file insurance claims and will schedule reasonable payment plans if necessary. If a private clinic has accepted your child as a patient and you later become unable to afford such care, that clinic has an ethical obligation to make sure that your child is referred to a public facility for care.

Take notes about your child's seizures and general health, as well as a written list of questions. Ask them first of the nurse, who is often the most appropriate person to provide such information. The best way to get a good start with your child's health care team is to show them that you are prepared to use their time wisely. While you are in the waiting room, review your notes to remind yourself of what you want to accomplish in the visit.

Also, be sure to ask your child if there is anything he would like to ask or tell the nurse or physician or other team member. Then, at an appropriate time during the visit, prompt your child to ask the question or share information. By continuing to actively involve your child to the extent of his abilities, you can build a sense of self-esteem and feeling of being an important member of the team. This also helps prepare the child for independence later in life.

If you are taking your child back for a routine clinic visit, expect to spend about fifteen to twenty minutes. Again, make a list of questions, and ask the nurse or nurse-clinician which ones he can answer and which ones to ask of the physician. When the physician comes in to see your child, mention that you have a few questions to ask when it is convenient.

You should not hesitate to talk with your child's physician, but don't feel free to chat at length about things that are not directly related to your child's health. Try to be as brief and as clear as possible when volunteering information. If a family member or friend can explain things better, ask that person to accompany you and your child. Your physician will appreciate any information that can improve your child's epilepsy control and general health. Be a good listener, and expect the physician to listen well in return. If the physician is using terms you do not understand, ask for an explanation. Repeat in your own words what you are hearing; this will tell the physician that you have understood important information.

What If Things Don't Work Out?

Many people find it difficult to ask a physician for a referral to another physician. Whether for a second opinion, for specialty care, or to change physicians, it is common to feel awkward, as if this request is a criticism of the physician's ability. There is no need to feel that way if you are convinced that your child's health care could be improved by seeing another physician. Medical ethics require physicians to refer patients for a second opinion if they are asked to do so.

As in any human relationship, sometimes a parent or child simply cannot communicate well or feel comfortable with a certain physician. Whatever the reason for wanting to take your child elsewhere, you need only express your desire to the physician or nurse. Try to be matter-of-fact in stating your request, without being judgmental or hostile. Perhaps if you explain to the nurse what type of personality you would feel more comfortable with, your child could be referred to another physician at the same clinic. If presented honestly and politely, your request will almost certainly lead to a referral to a respected health care team.

Are You Making the Most of the Nurse?

Nurses are often the "glue" that holds the health care team together. They can skillfully perform a variety of health-screening tests and procedures, and they gather much of the information the physician needs to make decisions. Nurses must also be skilled at communicating medical information to patients and family members, and they must make sure that the physician's instructions are understood.

One part of the nurse's job is to help you make the most of the time your child spends with the physician. To do that, the nurse needs your help and cooperation. Tell the nurse the reason for your visit and express any special concerns of which you want to be sure the physician is aware. Tell the nurse if you have a question or remember something else you wanted to ask after the physician sees your child. Your question will be addressed as soon as possible. However, if it is a major but nonemergency problem, you may have to make another appointment.

What Can the Nurse-Clinician Do for You and Your Child?

Some clinics employ nurse-clinicians, registered nurses who have special training in a specific area of medicine. The nurse-clinician can provide much of the routine care and exams usually done by physicians, freeing them to deal with more complicated problems.

The nurse-clinician can spend more time with your child and can answer many of your questions. The physician works closely with the nurse-clinician to determine what needs to be done at each visit and what changes, if any, need to be made in your child's epilepsy control plan. Time will be wasted if the nurse-clinician has to pry information out of you. By providing all the information the nurse-clinician asks for, you and your child will be assured of a successful visit.

The nurse-clinician is also a good resource when phoning the clinic with problems or questions about epilepsy. It is rarely necessary to speak to a physician about routine questions if a qualified member of your child's health care team is available. The nurse-clinician will either provide a solution, consult with the physician and call you, or have the physician return your call if necessary.

Who Else Is on Your Child's Health Care Team?

There may be several other members of your child's health care team who can help improve your child's seizure control and general well-being. A pharmacist, for example, can do more than fill prescriptions. Questions about epilepsy medications, side effects, interactions with over-the-counter medications, dosages, and generic versions of brand-name drugs may all be addressed by your pharmacist. (But *never* make any changes in your child's medications without first consulting your child's physician.)

Social workers and psychologists are often helpful because epilepsy affects all aspects of a child's life and the life of the family. By getting help before financial or emotional problems become severe, you can greatly decrease the stress and harmful impact felt by your child, yourself, and others you love. These professionals and a few others are discussed in later chapters. The most rewarding and enjoyable aspect of being a health care professional is helping patients and their family members who want to do everything possible to get the most out of life. By conveying that spirit and attitude, you and your child will become real members of the team and greatly improve the quality of care. By showing your child and everyone else that your goal is for him to live well with epilepsy, you motivate everyone to do their best to help make that happen.

CHAPTER 8

THE IMPORTANCE OF EARLY AND ACCURATE DIAGNOSIS

Epilepsy is a complex disorder. There are several different types of seizures a child can have, and there are specific ways to treat each type of seizure or combination of seizure types. Just because a child has a seizure does not necessarily mean the child has epilepsy. If your child does have epilepsy and is therefore likely to have more seizures, it is important to start treatment as early as possible.

The diagnosis of epilepsy can sometimes be made quickly and with confidence that it is accurate. This is especially true if the physician has a good description of the child's seizure (or has witnessed the child having a seizure) and if the problem fits a recognized syndrome. If proper treatment is prescribed, the child has no more seizures, and a brain problem requiring specific treatment does not exist, then all is well.

However, often the diagnosis is not clear or a treatment does not prevent additional seizures. If this is the case for your child, it is important that additional diagnostic tests be done. These tests may show that she does not have epilepsy or they may give your physician the information necessary to prescribe an alternative treatment that prevents seizures and allows your child to function normally. This chapter describes tests used to evaluate a child suspected of having epilepsy, as well as various other tests that may be used to discover more about a child's epilepsy.

Your Input Is the Important First Step

You, your child, and anyone else who witnesses your child's first seizure are quite likely to be distressed by the experience. It may be difficult to remember exactly what happened. Some witnesses may remember or describe events differently. However, any and all descriptions you, your child, or other witnesses can give about the child's feelings and behavior before, during, and after the seizure will be helpful. In fact, this is usually the most useful information. The physician will be especially interested in the following questions, which can help in classifying the type of seizure:

- ✦ Did the seizure begin in one part of the body?

- ✦ Did the child lose consciousness during the seizure?

- ✦ Did the child seem to lose awareness but not have any repetitive, confused, or aimless behavior?

- ✦ Did the child behave in an unusual manner before experiencing repetitive movements or other uncontrolled motions?

- ✦ Was the child confused or sleepy, or did she complain of a headache after the seizure?

If your child's seizure was severe, causing convulsions or unconsciousness, she probably was admitted to the hospital for one to three days for observation and testing. If the child's seizure was not severe enough to require hospitalization or if the hospital was not equipped to do extensive neurologic testing, your child's physician may decide on hospitalization for care and diagnostic testing. In the hospital, antiepileptic medication may be prescribed to avoid the potential danger of further seizures. If medication is not started immediately, the child should be supervised especially closely.

The first part of the diagnostic process is to obtain a complete medical history for both the child and the family. If epilepsy runs in the family, information about other affected relatives will help in diagnosing and treating the child. A physician or nurse taking the history may ask questions about the child's behavior, problems with bed-wetting, history of head injury, health problems as an infant, family health problems, mental health, and use of alcohol, street drugs, or medications.

Questions asked in a medical history may not be specifically related to epilepsy because it is important to know about the child's overall health and development. Nonepileptic causes of seizures may be suggested by the medical history. Accurate and complete answers to all questions can help an experienced physician to reach a complete diagnosis. Withholding any information out of fear or embarrassment severely reduces the chances of making an accurate diagnosis and preventing further seizures.

After the medical history, the physician performs a complete physical examination. Blood and urine may be taken for laboratory tests to see if the child has an infection or imbalance of minerals, blood glucose, or medication that could cause seizures.

A special effort will be made to evaluate the child's nervous system. Several different tests may be used to examine the nerves and brain. After the physical evaluation, the physician may decide to use one or more types of diagnostic technology to evaluate your child.

An EEG Records Brain *Function*

The test most commonly used to diagnose epilepsy is electroencephalography, usually abbreviated EEG. The EEG detects the very small electrical charges given off by different parts of the brain as it functions.

The EEG records brain electricity as a set of wavy lines, much like those generated by a seismograph during an earthquake. A neurologist can tell from the pattern of the recording if there is something wrong with a part of the brain. The recording is called an electroencephalogram, usually referred to as an EEG. The EEG recording often looks normal unless the child has had a seizure during the recording session.

Most initial EEG sessions last about thirty minutes, but additional recordings may be done for several hours or even for days in the hospital or with portable EEG equipment. If the seizures occur many days apart, it may be difficult to gain enough information from the EEG to allow for a complete and accurate diagnosis. Therefore, a normal EEG recording does not rule out epilepsy as the cause of a child's seizures. It may be necessary to have several EEG sessions of different lengths while your child is asleep, awake, and very tired.

Having an EEG is safe and virtually painless. It may appear threatening to a child, however, so it is helpful to prepare her by explaining the machine and the test in easily understandable terms. It is important that the child be able to relax physically and emotionally during the recording, so it may help to bring something comforting or distracting, such as a favorite stuffed animal or book. The only slight discomfort involved is when wires called electrodes are attached to the child's scalp. There is a slight rubbing or scraping when each electrode is attached. The technologist doing the test may ask the child to breathe rapidly at times and may shine a blinking light into the child's eyes. Ask your physician if there is a booklet that you can read to your child about having an EEG examination.

CT and MRI Scans Record Brain *Structures*

Two types of medical technology may be used to evaluate the structures of the brain. The first is called *computed tomography*, or

CT scanning (sometimes called a CAT scan). The CT scanner is a large machine that has a round opening for the patient's head. An X-ray camera inside this opening revolves around the patient's head, taking many pictures at different angles and depths. These are then assembled by a computer into composite images that show structures within the brain.

A CT scan is painless, but the child must remain as still as possible. The entire session takes about fifteen minutes, but it is only during periods of several seconds that the child must be still. A fluid called a contrast medium is sometimes used to produce better X-rays of blood vessels in the brain. There may be pain, similar to that felt when having an injection, when the needle is placed in a vein in the arm.

A radiologist examines the pictures after the CT scan is completed and the X-rays are assembled into pictures of the brain. This physician may be able to detect damage inside the brain that could be causing abnormal electrical signals that may be triggering seizures.

MRI, or *magnetic resonance imaging*, is a newer and much better technology than CT for epilepsy diagnosis. The MRI machine looks a lot like a CT machine. It uses a huge magnet to create a magnetic field within the patient's body. The magnetic field allows a computer to generate a picture of thin sections of the body. The computer assembles these slices to create more detailed pictures of structure than those produced by a CT scan. An MRI is now the test of choice for evaluating patients with epilepsy, as a CT scan is not sensitive enough to detect many conditions.

When Should More Diagnostic Testing Be Done?

There are several reasons for continuing to perform diagnostic tests or for repeating tests. If a child's seizures are not controlled by drug therapy after about three months, more tests should be done. If one is not already being consulted, this is also a good time to involve an epileptologist, a pediatric neurologist, or a neurologist who specializes in epilepsy.

The epileptologist may want to repeat some tests or to perform others. Children experiencing seizures can be especially hard to diagnose, so extensive testing is sometimes required. The physician will try to determine what type of seizure your child is experiencing. Some children have more than one type of seizure, and further diagnostic testing may be necessary to distinguish them. Knowing more about your child's seizure type or types will help the physician evaluate your child's medication and possibly to prescribe a more effective drug or combination of drugs.

If your child is still experiencing seizures one year after starting to take antiepileptic medications, she should be evaluated at a specialized epilepsy center, preferably a comprehensive epilepsy program, even earlier if possible. Physicians at such a center are most likely to be familiar with very recent discoveries about epilepsy diagnosis and treatment. They will reevaluate the results of the earlier diagnostic tests and your child's medication therapy. Specialized diagnostic tests may be done to clarify the diagnosis, and new medication therapy may be tried.

The epileptologist may decide to hospitalize your child for intensive neurodiagnostic monitoring. Most epilepsy centers work with a hospital that has special facilities to care for and monitor epilepsy patients with special combined video and EEG equipment. This method is most likely to record a seizure and provide the best information to the physician. When a seizure is recorded, the physician can match the behavior seen on video with the brain activity recorded in the EEG. Antiepileptic medications may be withdrawn during hospitalization to make it more likely that a seizure can be recorded.

If it is unlikely that a child's seizures will occur in the hospital, a method called ambulatory monitoring may be tried. This is used when seizures occur infrequently or only when the child is at home, at play, or in school. The child wears a small, portable EEG recording device connected to scalp electrodes. When the child feels a seizure about to begin, she pushes a button to mark when the seizure took place on the EEG recording. This method can be useful, but it is less effective than other means of EEG recording because the scalp electrodes often lose contact and a child is not always able to push the button to mark the seizure.

Computerized outpatient EEG monitoring is a new form of ambulatory monitoring that is far more useful. It can record more EEG channels and a computer can store recordings of seizure activity or other suspicious events. The computer can also reformat the EEG to help the epileptologist locate the origin of the seizures.

One group of tests that may be performed is known as a *neuropsychological examination*. These tests examine how different parts of the brain are performing and can help localize any disease or disorder that may be present. Some of these tests study motor function (body movements), reaction time, planning abilities, memory, and brain function.

An even newer technology is called *positron emission tomography*, or PET scanning. It looks at the metabolism of different parts of the brain, creating pictures by monitoring the use of oxygen and blood glucose by brain cells. This technology is used mostly in evaluating certain patients for epilepsy surgery and is available at some specialized epilepsy centers. Your physician may prescribe sedation to help your child rest quietly during the examination.

As you can tell by these descriptions of diagnostic tools for epilepsy, diagnosis can be a long and frustrating process, especially for children and their parents. However, epilepsy must be diagnosed properly in order to treat it properly. Good teamwork involving a cooperative family working with caring health professionals familiar with epilepsy diagnosis and treatment can be very rewarding. This team can work toward the ultimate goal: helping a child live well with epilepsy and grow into a happy, healthy, productive adult.

CHAPTER 9

ANTIEPILEPTIC MEDICATIONS: THE FIRST CHOICE TO CONTROL EPILEPSY

Epilepsy can rarely be cured, but it can usually be controlled. Epileptic seizures rarely go away on their own, but they can be prevented or at least drastically reduced with medication. That is why medications are the first choice when it comes to controlling a child's epilepsy.

Fortunately, there is a wide choice of medications that will prevent seizures in most children, and every year scientists discover new ones that control certain types of seizures better and with fewer side effects. The challenge in epilepsy control is to find the right antiepileptic medication (AED) or combination of medications in the right dosage to best control the seizures. Again, success depends on good teamwork involving health professionals and your family.

How Will Our Child's Physician Know Where to Start?

As explained in Chapter 8, the proper diagnosis of the type (or types) of seizures a child is experiencing is the most important step toward good seizure control. Certain AEDs are used to prevent certain types of seizures because the medications affect the brain in different ways, and sometimes in more than one way at the same time. Some medications increase the person's seizure threshold; others limit the spread of the seizure in the brain by slowing the electrical transmissions between nerve cells. Still others increase the ability of certain nerve cells to transmit signals that inhibit the spread of abnormal electrical activity during a seizure.

Although there are more than twenty AEDs available, some are used more often than others (see Table 9.1). Your child's physician will probably start with one of the most commonly used AEDs for your child's type of seizures. In addition to seizure type, other factors to be considered are: (1) any previous allergic reactions the child has experienced when taking medications; (2) the child's age, weight, and special physical problems; and (3) cost and your ability to pay.

Many physicians begin by prescribing a dosage somewhat less than the recommended daily dose (the amount that is known to be safe and effective for most children the same age and weight as your child). It can take a few days for the medication to reach a "steady state" level in the blood, so that the amount of drug the child is taking is about the same as the amount being eliminated. If your child tolerates this dosage but continues to have seizures, the physician may gradually increase the dosage until a safe and effective dosage is reached.

Some AEDs are taken once a day while others must be taken several times a day. This is because medications have different "half-lives," the time it takes for half of the dose to be eliminated from the body. A medication that is removed from the body more slowly can be taken less often than one that is removed more rapidly. It takes an average of five half-lives of a medication to reach steady state. However, children of the same age and weight can eliminate the

TABLE 9.1   Preferred Antiepileptic Medication by Seizure Type

Seizure Type	First Line	Second Line	Contraindicated
Generalized absence	Zarontin® Depakote®		Phenobarbital Mebaral® Mysoline®
Generalized tonic-clonic	Dilantin® Tegretol® Depakote®	Phenobarbital Mysoline® Felbatol® Lamictal® Neurontin®	
Tonic drop attack	Felbatol® Depakote® Klonopin®		Phenobarbital Mebaral® Mysoline®
Partial simple	Dilantin® Tegretol® Phenobarbital	Klonopin® Lamictal® Neurontin® Mysoline®	
Complex partial	Dilantin® Tegretol® Felbatol® Lamictal® Neurontin®	Phenobarbital Mysoline® Depakote® Klonopin®	
Secondarily generalized tonic-clonic	Dilantin® Tegretol® Felbatol® Lamictal® Neurontin® Depakote®	Phenobarbital Mysoline® Klonopin®	

N.B.   All medications can cause hypersensitivity reactions. Some have a relatively higher incidence than some of the other antiepileptic medications. Ask your physician to prescribe the safest *effective* medication for your child. It is better to take the small risk of aplastic anemia than to have severe uncontrolled seizures.

same medication from their bodies at different rates, depending on each child's individual metabolism.

The prescribed dosage will be the amount of the medication and the time or times it must be taken in order to keep a steady state level in your child's body. Your child's physician will tell you how much of the prescribed medication to give your child and when to give it. Be sure you understand this information, and write it down so you don't forget.

The effectiveness of all medications, including those for epilepsy, varies from one individual to another. Therefore, when medication therapy is begun, it is especially important to evaluate whether it is effective. Effectiveness is measured by two factors: (1) does it prevent seizures? and (2) does the child experience side effects?

A key factor in evaluating any medication's effectiveness is whether it was taken exactly as prescribed. With children, it is especially important to set up an easily remembered system for taking the medication.

Try to make taking the medication part of a daily routine, such as waking up and going to bed or at mealtimes, depending on how many doses are prescribed and at what intervals. Mark on a calendar when each dose is taken, and use a pillbox with compartments for each day's medication.

Ask your physician what to do if your child misses a dose. It is usually acceptable to give the missed dose as soon as you remember or to combine it with the next dose. It is NOT acceptable to skip the dose completely because this might reduce the amount of medication in the child's body to below the level needed to prevent seizures. By keeping tablets or capsules in a pillbox with compartments for each day, you and your child can check at bedtime to make sure the daily dosage has been taken. For liquids, reserve a place for the bottle to be kept before the medication is taken and another place to put it afterwards.

Watch your child closely to see if any side effects occur while taking a new medication or an increased dosage. Antiepileptic medications are quite safe when taken properly, but like all medications they may cause allergic reactions or other problems in some children. When the physician increases the dosage of a medication to try to obtain seizure control, it may reach a level in the child's body at which it causes unpleasant side effects.

Discuss with the physician what types of side effects your child might experience. See Table 9.2 for a list of common side effects caused by some antiepileptic medications. Most people do not have any of these side effects, and no one would have most or all of those listed. Notify the physician if you notice any of these side effects or if you notice anything unusual about the child's behavior or health.

TABLE 9.2   Side Effects of the Most Commonly Used Antiepileptic Medications

Drug	U.S. Trade Name	Common Side Effects with Monotherapy
Carbamazepine	Tegretol®	Sedation, diplopia, diarrhea
Clonazepam	Klonopin®	Sedation, dizziness
Ethosuximide	Zarontin®	Drowsiness, hyperactivity, nausea
Felbamate	Felbatol®	Insomnia, headache, weight loss, nausea, dizziness
Gabapentin	Neurontin®	Drowsiness, fatigue, dizziness, ataxia
Lamotrigine	Lamictal®	Diplopia, drowsiness, headache, nausea
Mephobarbital	Mebaral®	Drowsiness, lethargy, dizziness
Phenobarbital		Drowsiness, lethargy, dizziness, hyperactivity
Phenytoin	Dilantin®	Disturbance of equilibrium, hirsutism, gingival hyperplasia, acne, anemia, double vision
Primidone	Mysoline®	Drowsiness, appetite loss, irritability, nausea, vomiting, dizziness, loss of coordination, tremor
Valproic acid	Depakene® Depakote®	Indigestion, nausea, increased appetite, sedation, dizziness, hair loss, tremor, diarrhea

Side Effects

Side effects related to unacceptably high levels can be reduced by dividing the total daily dosage into more frequent smaller doses and by taking the dose with meals or at bedtime.

Side effects related to hypersensitivity are not dose-related and are largely unpredictable. They include:

- ✧ Rash
- ✧ Blood dyscrasia including aplastic anemia
- ✧ GI symptoms, especially diarrhea
- ✧ Drug-induced systemic lupus erythematosus
- ✧ Immunological disorders
- ✧ Lymphadenopathy
- ✧ Liver failure

It is usually possible to eliminate the side effect by reducing the dosage or changing the schedule.

There are two general causes of side effects: (1) too high a dose, and (2) allergic or hypersensitivity reactions.

Side effects related to too high a dose may include drowsiness, confusion, difficulty in thinking, loss of balance or muscular coordination, dizziness, hyperactivity, slurred speech, hiccups, muscle spasms, and eye twitching. Drowsiness and stomach problems can often be lessened by giving smaller doses more frequently or by giving the dose with meals or at bedtime. If problems persist, the physician might reduce the dosage to a lower level or substitute another medication.

Allergic or hypersensitivity reactions to antiepileptic medications are much less common than side effects caused by too high a dose. Symptoms might include rash, nausea, vomiting, diarrhea, severe drowsiness, mental confusion, and temporary kidney or liver dysfunction. Your child's physician will probably switch your child to another medication if these reactions occur.

The more severe hypersensitivity reactions to any kind of medication are most common in the blood system. Blood abnormalities of all sorts, including anemia, low platelet count, and low white count, can occur with many different medications. The problem usually reverses as soon as the medication is stopped. A low white count does not always require that medication be stopped. If your child really needs the medication, your physician can monitor the white count. At MINCEP® Epilepsy Care, we believe that as long as the child has at least 1,000 polymorphic nucleocytes, the absolute white count does not matter very much.

Aplastic anemia is by far the most dangerous of the hypersensitivity reactions. This can be seen with any medication. When Tegretol® was first introduced twenty-five years ago, there was an enormous scare about aplastic anemia caused by Tegretol®. Now we know that it occurs quite infrequently, and physicians prescribe Tegretol® freely to patients when it is helpful. Felbatol® was introduced in the summer of 1993, and on August 1, 1994, the Food and Drug Administration issued a warning because of what appeared to be a higher incidence of aplastic anemia with Felbatol® than with many other medications. At the time of this writing, the risk appears to be about 1 per 3,000–5,000 patients per year. This is enough to recommend caution in prescribing Felbatol®. However, Felbatol® is a very effective medication and if it controls your child's seizures when no other medication does, it is generally worth the slight risk of aplastic anemia against the certainty of severe uncontrolled seizures. Felbatol® also may, rarely, cause liver failure.

Aplastic anemia is recognized by a rash that looks like a cluster of little red dots, usually on the instep and the lower legs, easy bruising, severe fatigue, or severe infection. It is diagnosed by doing a blood count and seeing that the red and white count and the platelet count are low. If diagnosed early and treated properly, the majority of patients with aplastic anemia recover without any problems. Some require extensive, expensive treatment such as bone marrow transplantation. A few people, however, will die.

Write It Down!

A diary is an important tool in evaluating a medication's effectiveness. Until your child's seizures are under control, keep a complete record of when doses are taken and write detailed descriptions of any seizures or side effects that occur. Include time of day and what the child was doing when the seizure or side effect occurred. Do not try to memorize this information! Write it down in detail and take it with you when your child sees the physician. It can be a vital asset to good epilepsy therapy.

What If the Child's Seizures Continue?

Most children's seizures should eventually be controlled by one medication, although not necessarily the first one tried. Each medication and dosage level must be given adequate time to build up to an effective level; this sometimes takes as long as a few weeks. With a detailed diary and honest reporting of missed or delayed doses, you and your child's health care team can find the best medication or medications for your child.

During the time a new medication is being tried or the dosage increased, laboratory tests can be done to measure the amount of medication in your child's body. Since each individual metabolizes medications somewhat differently, it may be necessary to perform these blood tests frequently to help the physician evaluate the level of medication maintained in your child's body.

As the physician increases the dosage, your child may experience side effects from having too much of the substance in his or her system. This level, which is called "toxicity," is different for everyone. If your child reaches this level without having any reduction in seizures, the physician should begin substituting a second medication while slowly withdrawing the child from the first. The second medication will then be evaluated at gradually increasing dosages, just as the first one was.

If your child's first medication reduced seizures somewhat before reaching toxicity, the physician will probably add a second medication. Your child will continue to take the first medication, but at a dosage level below that at which toxicity occurred. If seizures continue, the physician will increase the dosage of the second medication until seizures are controlled or toxicity is reached. Frequent laboratory tests will be done during this process to evaluate how the two medications interact with each other. Seizure control can be achieved by most children with epilepsy through the proper use of just one medication. If a second one is added and is effective, the physician will gradually withdraw the first medication, unless seizures recur. The goal of medication therapy is to first control seizures without side effects, and then to achieve the simplest possible dosage regimen.

However, some children experience more than one type of seizure, or they may be unable to tolerate adequate levels of just one medication. These children can usually be helped by taking two medications. In rare cases of seizures that are especially difficult to control, it may be necessary for a child to take more than two medications.

As you and your child's health care team work toward finding the medication therapy that is best for your child, keep in mind the following success factors:

✧ Your child must take the right medication at the right time.

✧ Your child's blood levels must be checked appropriately.

✧ You must keep good records of your child's seizures and side effects.

✧ An experienced epilepsy team can help you and your child live well with epilepsy.

Can Epilepsy Medications Affect Other Medications?

Check with your child's physician before giving the child any other medications, including those that do not require a prescription. Seizure control is not affected if the child occasionally takes aspirin, acetaminophen (Tylenol®), or cold medications. To be safe, ask your physician or pharmacist before buying over-the-counter medications or when other medications are prescribed for your child. For example, some antibiotics given for ear infections or other bacterial infections, especially erythromycin, can double or triple the effect of some antiepileptic medications. Obviously, these types of interactions should be avoided if possible.

Most children see many different health professionals for many reasons, including routine medical care, dental checkups, and possible emergency treatment. Be sure to tell these health professionals that your child has epilepsy and is taking antiepileptic medication. A medical identification bracelet can help to convey this information when you are not present.

Can Epilepsy Medications Affect My Child's Teeth and Gums?

If your child is taking Dilantin® (phenytoin), inform your dentist and ask for special instructions regarding dental hygiene. Dilantin® is one of the oldest, safest, most effective, least expensive, and most commonly used antiepileptic medications. However, it causes swelling, overgrowth, and irritation of the gums in about one-fourth of the people who take it.

Good dental habits (which are a good idea anyway) can prevent the dental side-effects of Dilantin®. First, make sure your child follows a comprehensive dental care program, with regular cleanings, filling of cavities, and use of sealants and fluoride treatments. Daily dental care should include careful removal of food particles and prevention of plaque buildup. Try to avoid giving your child foods that stick to the teeth or between teeth. Carefully brush and floss your child's teeth when he is young, and teach the following dental care skills when he is older:

1. Use a soft toothbrush.

2. Hold the brush at a 45 degree angle to the teeth.

3. Wiggle the brush slightly, beginning at the base of each tooth, and bring it up toward the top of the tooth. Do not brush sideways.

4. Brush the tops of the teeth with the tip of the brush.

5. Include gums in up-and-down strokes to massage the gums and make them firm and resistant to irritation.

6. Brush the inside surface of teeth (near the tongue) and outside surface of all teeth, being especially careful to reach those at the back.

7. Use dental floss to clean the remaining two sides of each tooth, where it presses against neighboring teeth. Gently insert the floss between the teeth, then pull it back and forth in a sawing motion until it reaches the gums. Do this twice, holding the floss along each side of each tooth.

8. Waterpicks are also useful way for removing food particles from hard to reach surfaces. Plaque that does not come off with the brush may be removed with soft wood stimulators (Stimudents®) or even a clean popsicle stick.

Can I Save Money by Buying Generic Medications?

Cost is one factor a physician considers in choosing an antiepileptic medication, and this is something to discuss with your physician. *Never change your child's medication—either the brand name or the dosage—without first checking with the physician who prescribed it.*

Generic medications cost less because they are often manufactured by companies that have not invested in the research, development, and regulatory approval of the medication. Major pharmaceutical companies invest millions of dollars in each medication they invent, patent, and test, and to gain approval from the Food and Drug Administration (FDA) to sell the medication. A U.S. patent expires seventeen years after it is issued, and then any company can manufacture and sell the invention.

In the case of medications, the FDA continues to monitor generic products to make sure they meet acceptable quality standards, but there can be differences between generic medications and the same medication made by the original manufacturer. For example, the way the medication is made into a tablet or capsule can sometimes affect the way the medication is released into your body. In 1987, the FDA issued a warning that one of the generic types of antiepileptic medications was failing to control seizures in people who had been well-controlled when taking the brand name of the same medication.

In recent years the FDA has increased its overseeing of generic pharmaceutical manufacturers and distributors, but there still can be differences between generics and brand names. There can also be differences between one batch of generic medication and another because a distributor may put the same label on batches made by different manufacturers. Both types of differences are allowed by law, and the medications are generally safe. However, in the case of some people with epilepsy, a slight difference in the way a medication is manufactured or released in the body can alter its effectiveness.

Discuss with your child's physician the best way to reduce the cost of medication. It is often acceptable to switch to a generic form, but such a change must be supervised by the physician. Never allow anyone but your physician to make any change in your child's medication. Even a pharmacist should check with the physician before making any change or substitution. Once your child's blood levels have been regulated, it is important to stay on pills from the same manufacturer.

You can help ensure that your child gets the right medication by keeping a card in your wallet or purse with all the current information on your child's epilepsy medication and other medications the child is taking. Also record in your diary or logbook the distributor's name and the lot number each time you purchase the medication. This can help resolve questions if your child experiences side effects or seizures.

Another way to save money is to find a pharmacy that offers the best price on your child's medication. If your physician prescribes a generic form, you should be able to purchase it at nearly half the cost of the brand-name medication. If the price difference at your current pharmacy is not significant, you should find a pharmacy that passes along more of the savings for generic medications. If you cannot find the generic form at a significantly lower price, it might not be worth switching from the brand name. Your epilepsy team can help you make decisions about reducing your medication costs, and they can probably recommend pharmacies in your area that have the lowest prices.

What If My Child Won't Take Medications on Schedule?

As children grow up, many routine things can cause power struggles with their parents. Taking epilepsy medication can result in such a struggle. Chapters 16 through 19 contain helpful hints from parents about how to handle these power struggles with children of various ages. In all cases, the strategy is based on clear communication about why the medication is important and why it must be taken at the prescribed times.

A recent international conference of epilepsy experts reported that from 30 percent to 50 percent of people with epilepsy do not take their antiepileptic medications as scheduled. This was thought to be a major reason for uncontrolled seizures and the resulting disability.

As a parent, you must bear the primary responsibility for making sure that your child takes medications as prescribed. There may be occasional times when a pill is missed or delayed, but if taking medications becomes haphazard rather than routine, you must seek help from your epilepsy team. If getting your child to take the medication becomes a battle, ask for suggestions about how to make it easier. Living well with epilepsy includes the psychological well-being of your family as well as the physical health of your child, and the two often go hand in hand. Seeking help with a problem at an early stage is easier than trying to reverse years of struggling and poor seizure control.

What If Medications Don't Stop My Child's Seizures?

It is understandable for a parent to be impatient as medications are tried and adjusted in an attempt to control a child's seizures. Remember that it can take up to three months to fully test each medication at different dosages, and it can take longer if your child experiences only rare seizures. Do your best to remain patient during this time, but remain active in keeping a detailed diary and working with your epilepsy team to evaluate each medication and resolve any problems that arise.

If your child continues to have seizures, your physician should continue to make medication adjustments, to test the child's blood levels frequently, and to consult with an epilepsy specialist. If your child continues to have seizures and your physician is not treating your child vigorously and cannot explain the logic used to plan the next step, you should ask for a referral to an epilepsy specialist at a comprehensive epilepsy program.

Comprehensive epilepsy programs employ several types of health professionals with a wide range of expertise in helping people live well with epilepsy. They include epileptologists who specialize in treating either children or adults, nurse practitioners and nurse educators who assist patients and families in carrying out the epilepsy care program, psychologists and counselors who help patients and families solve the emotional problems related to epilepsy or daily living, nutritionists who help plan a healthy lifestyle, and social workers who help with financial problems or other life struggles. All of these health professionals believe in the team concept of epilepsy care, and they see you and your child as the most important members of that team.

After meeting with you and your child to go over the details of your child's care, the physician at the epilepsy program may want to hospitalize your child to perform the extensive diagnostic tests described in Chapter 8. These tests may suggest a new medication strategy or other change in therapy. Epilepsy programs also offer the newest types of antiepileptic medications, and they can closely monitor and evaluate your child while introducing these changes.

Everything possible should continue to be done to control your child's seizures, but it is not always possible to eliminate seizures completely. An experienced epilepsy team can help your child achieve the best possible seizure control and can help everyone in your family cope with the stresses that epilepsy can impose on all areas of your life.

Medication is almost always the first choice in epilepsy control, but surgery is becoming an increasingly successful second option. Although surgery for epilepsy is not new, it should be performed only at centers with extensive experience in evaluating patients, in performing various types of surgery, and a good track record. Surgery is now performed regularly at major comprehensive epilepsy centers. It is helping a growing number of people who have not been helped by medications. Be sure your child is fully evaluated by an experienced team at a comprehensive epilepsy program before surgery is performed.

Working with Your Child's Physician to Withdraw Medications

If a child has been seizure-free for at least two years, some physicians believe it may be possible to try to discontinue medications. Ask the physician to evaluate whether your child's seizure control is an indication that medications are no longer necessary. To evaluate whether this is likely to be successful, a series of diagnostic tests will be completed to try to detect any abnormalities that would cause seizures if medication is withdrawn. If abnormalities show up on an EEG recording or in other neurological tests, it may be unwise and possibly dangerous to withdraw medications.

In no case should a child or family stop medications "just to see what would happen." This can result in life-threatening status epilepticus (see Chapter 11).

When withdrawing a child from antiepileptic medications, the physician prescribes increasingly smaller doses of the medication over several weeks. The child should be watched closely during this time by parents and others, and any seizure activity should be immediately reported to the physician. If seizures are going to resume, they will most likely occur within six months to one year after the medication is stopped. However, only about one-third of children are able to stop medications completely.

Making a decision to attempt withdrawal from medications is easier when the patient is a child under sixteen years of age than it is for an older teen or adult. It is unfortunate if a child has a seizure during withdrawal, but there is little risk of major social problems occurring as a result.

For example, if an adult who has been seizure-free for several years has an unexpected seizure, the result could be loss of a driver's license, insurance problems, employment difficulties, and long-term loss of self-confidence. Most seizure-free adults who are not having problems with medications decide that it is better to continue therapy than to risk such serious consequences.

The next chapter explains how patients are evaluated for their potential to be helped by surgery, and what types of surgery are effective in controlling seizures.

CHAPTER 1 0

SURGICAL OPTIONS
FOR CHILDREN
WITH EPILEPSY

As we learn more about the human brain and how it is affected by various injuries and disorders, surgical options increase and improve in safety and effectiveness. Epilepsy is a major example. Among the patients at MINCEP® Epilepsy Care who have had surgery after careful evaluation, about 90 percent show useful improvement. Some still have seizures, but they are less frequent or less dangerous. There continue to be some risks related to epilepsy surgery, but it is becoming a safer option for an increasing number of patients who are not helped by medications.

When Is Surgery an Option for a Child with Epilepsy?

Each patient must be considered individually and evaluated carefully to determine whether surgery is an option. This chapter explains general factors considered in evaluating a child's potential to be helped by surgery and describes some of the most common types of epilepsy surgery. This is only a starting point, however. If you are considering surgery as an option for your child, seek as much information as you can, especially from an *experienced* comprehensive epilepsy program and from parents of children who have had surgery for epilepsy. It may be worth a journey to an epilepsy center that has many years of experience and has performed hundreds of operations.

Surgery is the first choice for treating epilepsy when seizures are caused by a brain tumor or a head injury that can be surgically corrected. Sometimes a CT or MRI scan reveals a bone fragment, blood clot, or tumor that is affecting part of the child's brain. Surgery may be less risky than leaving these problems untreated. Improvements in surgical techniques have made it possible to repair many brain injuries and remove some tumors without seriously affecting the patient's brain function.

Surgery is also considered when a child continues to have frequent or severe seizures or unacceptable side effects six months to one year after beginning trials of antiepileptic medication. Surgery can be especially beneficial if diagnostic tests show that the child's seizures begin in a small part, or focus, in the brain. If further tests determine that this focus does not serve a vital function, such as speech or memory, the team may recommend that the focus be surgically removed.

Another type of surgery can be performed when a child's seizures start in one area and then spread rapidly throughout the brain. These types of seizures often cause dangerous falls and injuries. Their severity can usually be reduced by cutting part of the tissue that connects the two halves of the brain. This stops the seizure from spreading throughout the brain, and it may make it possible to prevent seizures with medication.

Neither of the generalities discussed here (surgery for brain injury or tumor and surgery for medically uncontrolled seizures) is a rule. Each child must be carefully evaluated for the potential to benefit from surgery. Then, given as much information as possible, it is up to the family to decide whether to proceed with the operation.

Surgery should not be rushed into, but neither should it be delayed unnecessarily. If a child has been injured by falling spells caused by seizures or is otherwise in physical or mental danger, surgery should be seriously considered and promptly undertaken if medically indicated and desired by the family.

Determining if a child is a candidate for elective surgery for epilepsy involves many established members of the epilepsy team and some new members. This decision should only be made at a specialized comprehensive epilepsy center. If the epilepsy team decides that surgery should be considered, the patient and parents meet with neurologists and neurosurgeons who specialize in epilepsy, as well as a neuroradiologist, who will direct imaging studies of the child's brain. A neuropsychologist may perform special diagnostic tests to detect any areas of brain damage. A counseling psychologist or psychiatrist may also work with the team to explore how the child and family feel about the surgical option and to prepare them for the stress of the procedure. A social worker may also become involved in helping the family through the many tests and procedures involved and in coordinating payment, temporary accommodations if necessary, and other concerns. Rehabilitation professionals may be needed to help the child recover from the surgery.

How New Is Epilepsy Surgery?

Although modern techniques of epilepsy surgery have advanced rapidly in the past two decades, the practice dates back to 1828, when Dr. Benjamin Dudley, a Transylvania University professor in Kentucky, reported successfully removing skull fragments and blood clots from the brains of people who experienced seizures as a result of head injuries. At that time, operating rooms were quite primitive, with no anesthesia or sterilization. Remarkably, all five of Dudley's patients survived and did well. Others were not as lucky: half of the patients died as the result of similar operations in the United States and Europe during the remainder of the nineteenth century.

Removal of brain tumors was first done successfully in 1884 by a German surgeon, Dr. Rickman J. Godlee. The patient's tumor was diagnosed by a neurologist, Dr. Hughes Bennett, using knowledge gained by German researchers studying the brains of animals. They found that convulsions could be caused in precise parts of the body by electrically stimulating parts of the brain. Bennett used this method to locate his patient's tumor by observing the signs and symptoms it caused.

The modern era of epilepsy surgery began in the 1950s, when electroencephalography was first effectively used to locate the focus of epileptic seizures. Dr. Wilder Penfield, a Canadian neurosurgeon, is considered the father of modern epilepsy surgery. He founded the Montreal Neurological Institute, where Dr. Herbert Jasper showed that EEG recordings could be used to locate the focus of a patient's seizures. Penfield was one of the first surgeons to reduce the severity of a patient's seizures by removing parts of the brain without damaging vital functions.

Where to Go for Surgery

Today epilepsy surgery is performed in specialized centers throughout the world. Increased knowledge about the brain and epilepsy and improved surgical technologies and postsurgical care have contributed to making surgery a reasonably safe and effective option for some people.

Not all hospitals that offer surgery are qualified to do so. If you are considering surgery as a treatment for your child, have an experienced comprehensive center perform the procedure. Your child will need a careful medical and psychological evaluation. Ask how long a center has been in existence, how many procedures they have performed, how many procedures they have performed of the type your child needs, their complication rate, their success rate, and the size and experience of the surgical team.

The National Association of Epilepsy Centers recommends that a center operate on at least twenty-five patients each year to maintain quality. The center you choose should offer a full range of services, not just routine temporal lobectomies.

Some epilepsy groups have a reputation for operating on almost anyone. Bigger is not necessarily better. It is especially important to know when *not* to operate.

There is no substitute for *carefully* evaluating any epilepsy program, especially a surgical epilepsy program.

What Are the Common Types of Epilepsy Surgery?

To understand the most common types of epilepsy surgery, it is necessary to be familiar with the types of seizures described in Chapter 3. Extensive diagnostic testing is usually performed to determine exactly what type or types of seizures a patient is experiencing. Specialized EEG tests and other brain function tests may also be done in the hospital. This information is crucial in evaluating a patient's suitability for surgery and in planning the operation. Two types of epilepsy surgery are most commonly performed.

Temporal Lobectomy

The most common type of epilepsy surgery is called an anterior temporal lobectomy. This involves stopping complex partial seizures by surgically removing the front part of one of the temporal lobes of the brain.

The brain has two halves or *hemispheres*. One is called the "dominant" hemisphere because it controls most of the person's sensory, memory, and language functions. Each hemisphere has a temporal lobe (a rounded division—"lobe"—on each side of the head near the temple—"temporal"). One of the temporal lobes, usually the left, has more control of speech and memory for words than the other and is therefore called the dominant lobe.

Combined video and EEG recording of seizures is almost always necessary to determine whether a child has complex partial seizures that originate from one temporal lobe. Location of a structural problem in the same portion of the same temporal lobe with MRI or PET imaging helps to confirm the potential for surgery.

Neuropsychologic studies help locate the parts of the brain that are not working normally, helping physicians decide where and what parts of the brain can be usefully and safely removed.

A *Wada test* (intracarotid sodium amytal test) can be done to determine which hemisphere of the brain is dominant. The test involves injecting an anesthetic into the arteries on each side of the head. When it is injected into the artery supplying the dominant hemisphere, the child is temporarily unable to speak or may have memory problems. This helps determine whether the affected temporal lobe can be removed without seriously damaging the child's speech and memory abilities.

Another test called a *cerebral angiogram* may be done at the same time as the Wada test. A special fluid is injected into an artery, and X-rays are taken as the fluid flows through blood vessels in the brain. This provides the surgeon with a picture of where the blood vessels are located in the child's brain.

If questions remain about the precise location of the seizure focus, it may be necessary to perform diagnostic testing using special EEG electrodes placed precisely in selected parts of the brain. This is necessary because sometimes the weak abnormal EEG signals given off during a seizure cannot be detected through the skull. The probes are placed in an operation before the actual surgery, usually done under local anesthetic (without putting the patient to sleep). A device called a stereotactic frame is placed on the patient's scalp and used to guide electrodes into parts of the brain to enable localized EEG recordings to be taken. Monitoring may continue for one to three weeks, and then the probes are removed in a simple and relatively painless procedure. If the epilepsy team and the family decide to proceed with surgery, the child is sent home to allow the brain to heal for a month or more before the operation.

If testing indicates that the child's focus is located close to portions of the brain that control speech, movement, or feeling, additional studies are necessary. This may involve an operation under general anesthesia (patient unconscious), during which an array (grid) of EEG electrodes is placed under the outer covering of the patient's brain. Called a subdural grid or subdural electrode array, this device is placed directly over the part of the brain that appears to be the seizure focus. The surgeon then closes the patient's scalp, leaving the grid in place for EEG recording in the hospital.

The patient is allowed to rest for a day and is then taken to a video/EEG recording suite. EEG recordings are taken while parts of the patient's brain are stimulated, and the patient is monitored to locate speech and movement "centers." Recording through the subdural grid continues until enough seizures have been recorded to indicate precisely which area of the brain is involved and whether it is advisable to attempt to surgically remove the focus. This may take a week or longer. A second operation is necessary to remove the subdural grid, and if the epileptologists and family have decided in favor of epilepsy surgery, the focal tissue is removed during the same operation.

In our experience, 70 to 90 percent of people who have a temporal lobectomy are seizure-free after surgery. About 50 percent are seizure-free and 75 percent are helped if a subdural grid or depth electrodes are needed. Many surgical patients must continue to take medications to control their seizures. There is approximately a 2 percent risk of complications with partial loss of motor function (muscles), memory, or speech after a temporal lobectomy. Death is a very rare complication.

Corpus Callostomy

The second most common type of epilepsy surgery involves partly disconnecting the two hemispheres of the brain in an operation called a *corpus callostomy*. The hemispheres communicate with each other through a bundle of nerve fibers called the corpus callosum. If a person has seizures that start in one hemisphere, the abnormal electrical activity may spread through the corpus callosum to the other hemisphere. These *generalized* seizures can be dangerous, causing the person to fall without warning. They are also resistant to control with medications, making such patients good candidates for surgery.

Some of the same preoperative tests are done in evaluating a patient for a corpus callostomy as are done for a temporal lobectomy. The major difference is that invasive EEG recording (placing EEG probes into the brain tissue using a stereotactic frame or placing a subdural grid) is not necessary in evaluating a patient for a corpus callostomy.

The corpus callostomy operation ordinarily involves cutting the front two-thirds of the corpus callosum. This often prevents or reduces the number of seizures that involve both hemispheres. The remaining nerve fibers of the corpus callosum are sufficient to allow the patient's hemispheres to function normally together. The patient usually continues to have partial seizures, but they are much less dangerous because they do not usually cause falls. Few patients who have a corpus callostomy are seizure-free after surgery, but most have less severe seizures that can be controlled with medications.

If dangerous generalized seizures continue, some patients may require a second surgery to completely separate the two hemispheres. This reduces communication between the two halves of the brain, but it is preferable to continuous falling injuries from seizures.

There is approximately a 2 percent risk of complication as a result of a corpus callostomy. Approximately 80 percent of our center's patients who have undergone this operation have improved seizure control.

Other Types of Epilepsy Surgery

Other types of epilepsy surgery are far less common than the temporal lobectomy and corpus callostomy. One type of surgery done in selected cases is a *hemispherectomy*. This surgery is performed when a young child has one badly diseased hemisphere, resulting in significant paralysis of one side of the body and many severe seizures daily. Fortunately, these children can often be successfully rehabilitated because of the amazingly resilient ability of the remaining hemisphere to take over much of the control of both sides of the body.

Other types of surgery are being studied as options for patients who cannot be helped by the more common operations. They are becoming possible because of animal research and through the improvement of technologies for imaging and studying the brain. Information on these surgical developments is available through comprehensive epilepsy programs.

Is Surgery an Option for Your Child?

If you are still unsure about surgery for your child after reading the preceding information and discussing your child's situation with your epilepsy team, request the names of other parents who have been through this experience. They may be better able to explain how their child tolerated the many diagnostic tests and operation(s).

Ask to speak to at least one family whose child has had a satisfactory outcome and at least one whose child has had a poor outcome. As with any major surgery, the patient and family must be prepared for all possible outcomes. Hearing how others have coped with the preoperative uncertainty and the postoperative rehabilitation can help you decide whether or not to proceed.

Include your child in these meetings and deliberations to the fullest extent of her ability to understand and participate. Share your hopes and feelings with your child and with other loved ones and friends. They can often provide the support and encouragement that will make any decision you make the right one.

One misjudgment that some people make about epilepsy surgery is to consider it the solution to all their problems. This places an unfair burden on everyone involved. The best that can be hoped for is that the child will be seizure-free or that seizures will be controlled with medication. Surgery cannot remove the stresses you and your child have already experienced, and there will likely be many challenges ahead. Talking with others who have experienced epilepsy surgery and a psychological counselor can provide valuable personal insights and a realistic outlook on these issues.

If you decide to proceed with surgery, make a pact to think and act positively in the time before the operation. This will help everyone, especially your child, to prepare for that day and to make the best of the outcome, whatever it might be.

What Will a Child Experience After Surgery?

Details of a patient's preparation for surgery and what will take place during surgery is provided by the team performing the operation. The operation usually takes several hours, after which the child is moved to a recovery area. After the anesthesia wears off, a few family members may be able to visit. The child may have facial bruising and swelling and will be very tired, possibly for several days. The average stay in the hospital after surgery is about a week, but this depends on the type of surgery and how the patient recovers. Some of the tests done before surgery are repeated afterward to evaluate the outcome. Rehabilitation begins in the hospital and a schedule of outpatient visits is set.

Recovery after temporal lobectomy usually takes a few weeks, during which the child may experience headaches and lethargy. It takes from six weeks to six months to fully recover from a complete section of the corpus callosum, during which time the child may be lethargic, irritable, and clumsy. Recovery from a partial section of the corpus callosum is usually much easier.

Remember that complete elimination of seizures without the use of medications is not a realistic outcome for most patients. Most patients have fewer and less severe seizures, and medications often bring the remaining seizures under control within one to two months after surgery.

No matter what the decision is about surgery to try to control a child's epilepsy, there is always hope. New medications and new procedures are continuously being developed and tested through research and clinical practice. By staying aware of this progress, you and your child can be ready to participate in the quest for a better future.

CHAPTER 11

FIRST AID
FOR SEIZURES

If you ask people what they think they should do if they witness someone having a seizure, some would probably say, "Put something in the person's mouth so they don't swallow their tongue." This misinformation has led to many broken teeth and bitten fingers!

As a parent of a child with epilepsy, you can help counter this popular misconception by helping to inform your family, friends, your child's teachers and babysitters, and the public about proper first aid for epileptic seizures. Although they may be reluctant and fearful at first, you can reassure them that very little intervention is necessary. In general, one should comfort the person having a seizure, remove dangerous objects, and call for emergency assistance if the seizure does not stop within a minute or two. There is information in the appendix that you can copy to give to them.

It Is Impossible to Swallow Your Tongue

The type of seizures most familiar to the public are generalized tonic-clonic seizures, in which the person may fall, stiffen, make jerking movements, and bite his tongue. The skin may turn pale or bluish because of difficulty breathing, which is probably where the notion about swallowing the tongue originates.

It is impossible to swallow your tongue, whether you are having a seizure or not. A person having a seizure may have difficulty breathing, but he is seldom in danger of suffocating *if properly assisted*. Putting something in his mouth only makes it harder to breathe. It can also cause broken teeth and an injured jaw for the person with epilepsy, and finger injuries for the misinformed giver of first aid.

Several simple first aid steps can be taken to help a person having a seizure. In general, remain calm and inform others witnessing the seizure what is happening and that you know what to do, unless one of them is more experienced with handling seizures. Do not try to shake the person out of the seizure or restrain him, and do not let anyone else try to jam something into his mouth. Simply remove any dangerous objects in the area and wait until the seizure is over.

Reassure the person during and after the seizure by speaking softly. If the seizure stops and the person regains awareness, it is usually not necessary to call an ambulance, unless he has been injured. Check for a Medic Alert bracelet for the telephone number of someone to call. If the person can communicate, ask if there is anything you can do to help or anyone you can call. Offer to help the person get home or to a physician and offer to provide a description of the seizure.

Following are some additional steps that can be taken, depending on which of three types of seizures the person is experiencing.

Generalized Tonic-Clonic Seizures

Tonic-clonic seizures are most familiar to the public because they are the most dramatic. The person may fall, stiffen, make jerking movements, turn bluish from uneven breathing, and lose control of the bladder or bowel. The person is unable to respond to anyone during the seizure and may be confused and sleepy afterward. The following are a few suggestions for offering assistance.

1. Help the person lie down and put something soft under the head. If children are present, tell them what is happening and assure them that the person having the seizure will soon be fine.

2. Remove eyeglasses and loosen any tight clothing (such as a tie or top button) if possible.

3. Clear the area of sharp objects, such as furniture.

4. *Do not* force anything into the person's mouth.

5. *Do not* try to restrain the person.

6. After the seizure, turn the person on one side in order to let saliva drain from the mouth and the tongue to fall forward and open the airway. It may be helpful to push the jaw forward after the shaking has stopped.

7. The person may be confused upon awakening. Calmly reassure him that everything is all right.

8. *Do not* give the person anything to eat or drink until he is fully awake.

9. Stay with the person until he is fully alert, then ask if there is anything you can do to help. Help him maintain as much dignity as possible by quietly offering a coat or other material to conceal any evidence of loss of bowel or bladder control and by helping the person to find a bathroom. This is especially important if a child has had a seizure in front of other children. Inform them what is happening, but help the child avoid as much embarrassment as possible by quietly and quickly helping him to a private area.

Complex Partial Seizures

Complex partial seizures are the most common type of seizure. The person usually appears to be awake but may speak nonsense or not respond. The person may have a glassy stare, respond incorrectly to simple questions or not at all, move about aimlessly, make lip-smacking or chewing motions, fidget with clothes, and become angry or aggressive if restrained. This behavior is sometimes mistaken for drunken or drugged behavior, which is another reason it can be helpful for a person with epilepsy to wear a Medic Alert bracelet or necklace. Here are a few suggestions for helping:

1. Do not try to restrain the person from wandering.

2. Remove harmful objects from the person's path, and gently coax him away from stairs or other hazards. Stop or restrain him only if absolutely necessary to prevent an accident. Get help if he is in danger.

3. Try to calm the person. *Do not* shake or shout at him.

4. After the seizure, the person may be confused. Stay with him until fully alert, then describe what happened and ask if there is any way you can help.

Absence Seizures

Absence seizures occurs mostly in children. Others may not notice them because the only outward sign may be rapid blinking or a blank stare. The child appears to be awake but is briefly unaware of surroundings and events. He may miss parts of a conversation or a school lesson or may have incomplete memories of recent events. The following are helpful suggestions:

1. Absence seizures are usually very brief, but if you notice that the person is unaware of surroundings, watch to see how long the seizure lasts and what he does during the seizure.

2. When the person regains awareness, provide any information he missed and help him get back into the lesson, conversation, or activity.

When Does a Seizure Become a Medical Emergency?

Most seizures last less than a minute or two, and the person usually does not require medical assistance. However, on rare occasions it may be necessary to call an ambulance. If the person is seriously injured during a seizure or does not start breathing within two minutes, call an ambulance and then begin to treat the injury or give mouth-to-mouth resuscitation. If the person seems fine and has regained awareness, ask him if you should call an ambulance or a physician.

It may also be necessary to call an ambulance if a tonic-clonic seizure does not stop after two or more minutes or if another seizure starts very soon after the first one ends. The person could be experiencing a condition called status epilepticus (continuous seizure state) that can be life-threatening and requires special treatment as quickly as possible.

What Causes Status Epilepticus?

A person is in danger of status epilepticus if antiepileptic medication is stopped suddenly or is not taken often enough to maintain effective blood levels. A less common cause is an illness with fever or infection, which can increase the metabolism and cause the body to eliminate medication too quickly to be effective.

Status epilepticus must be treated in the hospital, where the patient's breathing can be restored and the seizures stopped with intravenous medications. Blood tests should be done to find out what caused the episode. The patient must be watched carefully until the seizures have stopped, and then the physician who supervises his epilepsy therapy should be contacted.

We Must Educate the Public

Having a seizure can be embarrassing, especially when others respond inappropriately by creating a scene. Out of fear and misunderstanding, some children and even adults may ridicule or avoid the person with epilepsy after a seizure. The best way to help everyone is through public education about seizures.

Start by teaching your friends and relatives what to do when a seizure occurs. Emphasize that there is really very little to do except to reassure the person and make the area safe. Suggest that they help you to spread accurate information to others, and work with your child's school and epilepsy caregivers to teach children and adults about epilepsy and seizures.

We may soon be able to ask people what they think they should do for someone having a seizure, and hear refreshing responses such as: "I would just help the person avoid injury during the seizure and then offer to help in whatever way I could afterward."

CHAPTER 12

SEIZURES IN NEWBORNS

Seizures are not unusual at birth and during the first few weeks of life. They must be evaluated immediately and treated appropriately to prevent serious long-term disability or death. Fortunately, seizures in a newborn often can be quickly stopped by treating the cause. If a newborn has already had one or more seizures and is undergoing treatment, parents and other family members should learn to recognize symptoms and report them immediately to the physician.

What Could Cause a Newborn to Have Seizures?

Seizures in newborns are often caused either by complications during birth or by a chemical imbalance or infection in the days following. Because the baby's brain and brain function developed in the uterus, injuries to the brain before birth are also a major cause of seizures. After delivery, an imbalance of nutrients or an infection in the blood and spinal fluid can cause seizures. These causes of seizures must be immediately investigated, and proper treatment must be initiated quickly. This is especially true for premature babies.

Seizures may be caused by many different types of birth injuries. Problems present at birth are called *congenital disorders*. Some affect the brain directly, whereas others have an indirect effect. A newborn may have bleeding within the brain (intraventricular hemorrhage), blockage of blood flow in the vessels leading into the brain causing a stroke, or the brain may not receive enough oxygen.

Other congenital disorders may involve improper development of organs such as the heart, kidneys, and lungs. Improper function of these organs can cause chemical imbalances in the blood or can result in insufficient oxygen being delivered to the brain.

Sometimes a baby is born without the ability to make enough of one of the many types of chemicals that the brain needs to function. These disorders are "inborn errors of metabolism" that involve the basic ways in which body cells process nutrients.

A fairly common cause of newborn seizures is imbalance of minerals or dehydration (not enough body water) often as a result of vomiting or diarrhea. Lack or imbalance of other nutrients and enzymes can also cause seizures. Proper amounts of body water and many of the substances carried in the blood and urine are necessary to maintain normal function. Because they have a much smaller amount of blood and fluids, babies can develop shortages and imbalances much faster than children and adults. A physician can usually diagnose these imbalances by asking the parent about the baby's digestion and bowel movements and by testing blood and urine. Replacing missing fluids and nutrients usually prevents further seizures and restores health.

Another potential cause of seizure in a newborn is rapidly rising temperature caused by an infection, or by an infection in the brain. This is not a simple "febrile" (meaning feverish) seizure, which is most common in children between the ages of six months and four years (see Chapter 13). The cause of such seizures in newborns must be identified and treated, and steps must be taken to control the seizure. Seizures in newborns are not "epilepsy" as much as they are symptoms of underlying illness or disease requiring treatment.

What Do Seizures Look Like in Newborns?

Seizures in a newborn are often quite subtle, and it may be difficult to recognize the seizure activity as abnormal behavior. Newborns almost never have tonic-clonic convulsions, in which the body stiffens and then has rhythmic, jerky movements. The newborn's brain is not developed enough to support this type of generalized seizure. Instead, newborn seizures usually involve some type of repetitive, almost mechanical behavior.

The following behaviors may indicate that a newborn is having a seizure:

✧ Staring that cannot be interrupted by moving something in front of the baby's eyes;

✧ Unusual rhythmic movement of the eyes;

✧ Rhythmic movement of one or both arms or legs that continues when the baby is moved or the limb is held;

✧ Rapid flexing of the legs against the body;

✧ Sudden loss of body tone;

✧ Sudden jerky movements;

✧ Any behavior that cannot be stopped by holding, touching, or repositioning the baby.

A newborn should be immediately seen by a physician if any of these behaviors is detected. Many turn out not to be seizures, but in the first weeks of life it is especially important to carefully evaluate any sign of a congenital disorder or birth injury.

Sometimes behaviors during sleep are mistaken for seizures. These include frequent jerky eye movements during a period of deep sleep called "rapid eye movement" sleep, or irregular breathing or twitching during sleep. Other normal behaviors may appear to be similar to the behaviors described previously. Do not hesitate to ask your baby's physician or nurse about any behavior or appearance that seems unusual.

How Are Newborn Seizures Diagnosed?

A newborn suspected of having a seizure should be immediately evaluated through tests of urine, blood, and spinal fluid. A neurologic exam should also be conducted to evaluate the baby's awareness, alertness, and response to noise. However, it is difficult to detect many disorders because the baby's brain is not sufficiently developed. It is usually necessary to do an MRI scan to rule out any structural problem in the baby's brain.

EEG monitoring is useful in evaluating newborn seizures. It is usually done continuously for a day or two, rather than for a half hour or an hour as in older children and adults, because it is especially difficult to detect abnormal electrical activity in a newborn's brain as opposed to the normal patterns of electrical activity that reflect the baby's still developing brain. The recording should be read by a neurologist who is familiar with seizures and EEG recordings in newborns.

How Are Newborn Seizures Treated?

Treatment must be started immediately if a baby has continuous seizures. This emergency treatment includes helping the baby breathe, giving intravenous solutions of glucose and other nutrients, monitoring the baby's heart, and giving other antibiotics and medications as necessary. If seizures continue, the baby may be given phenobarbital, the medication used most commonly for newborn seizures. This emergency treatment is designed to prevent immediate danger to the baby and to reduce neurologic damage from the seizures.

Once the baby's seizures stop, the type of treatment used depends on whether the physician is able to detect a specific abnormality through diagnostic tests. Treatment must be started immediately if the seizure was caused by lack of body fluids or nutrients or by an infection.

If the EEG recording or the MRI scan reveals a problem in the brain, an antiepileptic medication may be prescribed to prevent additional seizures. The baby should then be referred to a pediatric neurologist for evaluation and continuing treatment.

A thorough evaluation by a pediatric neurologist is absolutely necessary before long-term treatment with antiepileptic medications is begun. Seizures must be prevented if at all possible, but it is also important to give the lowest dosage of medication that is effective, so that the baby is able to develop as normally as possible, both mentally and physically. Medications can often be discontinued after several months if no seizures occur and EEG recording is normal, but this must be done very carefully under the direction of a pediatric neurologist.

The most important thing to keep in mind about newborn seizures is that they must be evaluated immediately and treated quickly and effectively. In many cases, the underlying cause can be treated and the child will not be adversely affected and will not continue to have seizures that require treatment with antiepileptic medications.

If a congenital defect or birth injury is detected, there is a good chance that it can be treated. About half of the infants who experience seizures consequently have some type of health problem later in life, but many problems can be prevented by early and complete evaluation and effective treatment.

CHAPTER 13

SEIZURES IN INFANTS

As a baby outgrows the newborn stage, it is less common to see seizures caused by birth injuries or acute bacterial infections, although seizures can still be triggered by a variety of imbalances, disorders, and injuries that may take months to become apparent. Once the infant passes six months of age, two new types of "seizures" can occur: febrile seizures and breath-holding spells. As in newborns, any suspected seizure activity in an infant must be evaluated immediately and treated appropriately to prevent serious long-term disability or death.

Prevention Is the First Step

A significant cause of seizures and epilepsy during the first year of life is head injury. Parents are usually protective of a newborn, but despite their best efforts, infants are exposed to more risks as they begin to move about and explore their world. Infants may pull lamps and other objects onto themselves, may fall against hard or sharp objects, or may be dropped by older children. Sadly, some children experience serious head injury from abusive adults. Shaking an infant in anger can cause serious untreatable injury.

Far too many infants are not secured properly in approved seats when riding in cars or on bicycles. Accidents happen, but there is much that parents can do to prevent them. Make sure that the areas of your house the infant is exploring are safe, and do not let young children hold or carry an infant without close supervision.

If your infant has experienced seizures, be careful to prevent head injuries from normal or seizure behavior, but do not restrict the infant from developing normally by crawling, sitting, standing, and walking. If your infant experiences seizures as the result of a preventable accident, you can become a powerful force for educating other parents about preventing head injuries. You can also help your child overcome any resulting disability by promoting positive self-esteem and emphasizing what the child can do and learn.

What Causes an Infant to Have Seizures?

Seizures in infants may be caused by a chemical imbalance, dehydration, infection, fever, congenital disorders, reduced oxygen supply to the brain, or injury to the brain. A congenital disorder may become apparent only as the baby's brain and brain function develop. It is important to have well-baby checkups to make sure the infant is progressing normally in weight, size, and behavior.

Because the infant is still small, imbalances of nutrients, minerals, or important enzymes in the blood and spinal fluid can cause a seizure more easily than in older children and adults. These problems may occur if the baby was born with certain inborn errors of metabolism that only become apparent during the baby's rapid growth of the first year.

As an infant reaches two or three months of age, she begins to lose some of the immunity provided by the mother. Breast-feeding can prolong some of this immunity. However, all infants gradually become more susceptible to bacterial infections and viral illnesses that cause fever, lethargy, vomiting, and diarrhea. Seizures can result from the effect of these conditions on the brain. They can usually be treated quickly with medications, fluids, and supplemental nutrients and minerals.

Vomiting or diarrhea can cause an infant to lose too much body water, resulting in dehydration (not enough body water). An infant with vomiting or diarrhea for more than twenty-four hours should be seen by a physician. During the first few months, an infant may become dehydrated rather quickly. Signs of serious dehydration include lack of tears when crying, lack of normal drooling from the mouth, absent or reduced urination that is dark in color, sunken appearance around the eyes, and lethargy.

Another potential cause of an infant's seizure is rapidly rising temperature caused by an infection. "Febrile" (feverish) seizures are most common in children between the ages of six months and five years. About one in thirty children has at least one febrile seizure, and roughly half of those who have a febrile seizure have more than one. Febrile seizures are seldom dangerous in themselves, but they should be evaluated by a physician to determine the cause of the fever.

If the cause is a simple viral infection, the physician will probably recommend treating the seizure with a cool bath and acetaminophen (Tylenol®). A newborn who has one or a few febrile seizures will probably not have any resulting health or developmental problems, but treatment with antiepileptic medications may be necessary if they occur frequently. Children usually outgrow febrile seizures and medication can be discontinued under a physician's supervision. Febrile seizures tend to run in families. A family history of febrile seizures helps the physician make the diagnosis. When a child first has a seizure with fever, it is not always easy to determine whether it is a simple febrile seizure or the beginning of epilepsy.

As an infant reaches six months of age, he may begin to develop breath-holding spells that mimic seizures, but rarely produce one. These spells (also called apneic spells) are usually provoked by pain, anger, or frustration. The child may scream, cry, stop breathing, turn pale or perhaps blue before beginning to breathe and cry again. These spells can cause seizures if the brain is temporarily deprived of oxygen. The infant should be evaluated by a physician, but these seizures are seldom a sign of epilepsy. Parents can help a

child overcome these spells by watching for signs of what is causing the infant's behavior and by calming or reassuring the infant during these times.

What Do Seizures Look Like in Infants?

Seizures in an infant are usually more obvious than they are in
newborns because the infant's brain is more developed and muscle
control in the arms and legs is greater. Like newborns, infants rarely
have generalized tonic-clonic convulsions during which they stiffen
and then have rhythmic, jerky movements of the body. An infant's
seizures are more likely to consist of staring for minutes at a time
that cannot be stopped by moving something in front of the eyes,
and by repetitive and sometimes violent movements of the arms and
legs. Breathing may be uneven, causing the infant to turn pale or
slightly blue.

An infant's seizure seldom lasts more than three minutes. First
aid is similar to that for an older child or an adult. The infant should
be placed on her side to allow free breathing and should be
watched until the seizure ends. Do not try to restrain the infant's
movements or force something into the mouth. If the seizure continues longer than approximately three minutes, it may be necessary
to call for emergency assistance. Mouth-to-mouth resuscitation is seldom necessary in infants, but it is a good idea for any parent to learn
the proper technique for infants and children.

The following behaviors may indicate that an infant is having a
seizure:

✦ Staring that cannot be interrupted by moving something in
front of the baby's eyes;

✦ Unusual rhythmic movement of the eyes;

✦ Uneven breathing with pale or bluish skin;

✦ Rhythmic movement of one or both arms or legs that continues when the baby is moved or the limb is held;

✧ Rapid flexing of the legs against the body;

✧ Sudden loss of body tone;

✧ Sudden jerky movements;

✧ Any behavior that cannot be stopped by holding, touching, or repositioning the infant.

An infant should be seen immediately by a physician if any of these behaviors is detected. Many turn out not to be seizures, but the infant must be evaluated carefully and treated appropriately. Do not hesitate to ask your infant's physician or nurse about any behavior or appearance that seems unusual.

How Are Seizures in Infants Diagnosed?

Diagnosis begins when parents record how the infant looked and behaved just before, during, and after the suspected seizure behavior. This is important to allow the physician to distinguish between febrile seizures, breath-holding spells, and possible epileptic seizures. An infant suspected of having a seizure should be immediately evaluated through tests of urine, blood, and spinal fluid. A neurologic exam should also be conducted to evaluate the baby's awareness, alertness, and response to noise. As the infant grows older, it becomes easier to detect neurologic disorders by evaluating muscular function and coordination. It may be necessary to do an MRI scan to rule out any structural problem in the infant's brain.

EEG monitoring is useful in evaluating seizures in infants. It may be done for many hours at a time rather than for a half hour or an hour as in older children and adults. This is because it is especially difficult to distinguish between abnormal electrical activity in a infant's brain and the normal changing patterns of electrical activity as the brain develops. An infant's EEG should be read by a neurologist who is familiar with seizures and EEG recordings in infants.

How Are Seizures Treated in Infants?

Treatment must be started immediately if an infant is having continuous seizures (status epilepticus). This emergency treatment includes helping the infant breathe, giving intravenous solutions of glucose and other nutrients, monitoring the infant's heart, and giving other antibiotics and medications as necessary. The infant may be given lorazepam (Ativan®), phenytoin (Dilantin®), or phenobarbital—the medications most commonly used for infants with seizures. The purpose of this emergency treatment is to prevent immediate danger to the infant and to reduce neurologic damage from the seizures.

Once the infant's seizures stop, further treatment depends on whether the physician is able to detect a specific abnormality through diagnostic tests. If the tests indicate that the child had a febrile seizure or a seizure caused by lack of body fluids or nutrients, any infection must be treated and lost fluids and nutrients should be replaced. No treatment other than parental counseling is necessary for breath-holding spells.

If EEG recording or MRI scan reveals a problem in the brain, antiepileptic medication may be prescribed to prevent additional seizures. If it does not prevent seizures, or if the infant has side effects or her activity or alertness is lowered, she should be referred to a pediatric neurologist. It is extremely important to quickly accomplish the two objectives of seizure control in an infant: no seizures and no side effects. This helps the infant achieve the goal of normal growth and development.

A pediatric neurologist can help establish an accurate diagnosis of a child's seizures if they are not clearly related to fever, breath-holding, or a temporary illness. This specialist can also help to achieve a safe and effective medication dosage. The infant can then return to her pediatrician or family physician for routine care. The infant's primary physician can consult with the pediatric neurologist about changes in medication or dosage. Antiepileptic medications can sometimes be discontinued after several months if no seizures occur and EEG recording is normal, but this must be done carefully under the direction of a pediatric neurologist.

Many infants experience seizures that are not a sign of epilepsy. The temporary illness, imbalance, or behavior that caused the seizure can usually be quickly diagnosed and corrected. The key to protecting the infant's health is to carefully record behavior and appearance before, during, and after the seizure and to work with your physician and a pediatric neurologist to determine the cause and proper treatment if necessary.

It is important to try to completely control seizures in infants. Although infants are less likely than older children to break bones, seizures interfere with an infant's normal intellectual, motor, and social development. If a pediatric neurologist has not brought the seizures under complete control without side effects within six months, the infant should be referred to a comprehensive epilepsy program that has special facilities for children.

CHAPTER 14

SEIZURES IN CHILDHOOD

Seizures are not good for either a child's brain or his sense of self-image. It is therefore never acceptable to take a "wait and see" attitude with a child who has had one or more seizures of unexplained cause. The importance of early diagnosis and appropriate treatment to prevent seizures without causing side effects cannot be overemphasized. Early intervention and involvement of the child and family with an epilepsy center can help achieve the best possible seizure control and prevent problems later in life.

This chapter discusses some of the special concerns parents have about treating a child's seizures. Remember, however, that seizure control is just one part of successfully living with epilepsy. A child and family will have many other challenges and concerns. These concerns and practical tips for parents are included in Chapters 16–19.

Prevention Is the Best Therapy

A significant cause of childhood seizures and epilepsy is head injury. Automobile accidents, bicycle and skating accidents, falls from playground equipment, rough play in the home, and sports

injuries can cause head injury, as can abusive adults and street violence.

Many, but not all, head injuries can be prevented. There are
several rules. Children *must* use a car seat approved for their age or
a seatbelt when riding in a car. Children *must* wear a helmet when
bicycling, skating, or riding horseback. Young children *must* be
supervised on playground equipment. Children *must* be restrained
from running or rough play in the home. Everyone playing sports
must wear appropriate protective equipment and learn how to play
the sport safely. And every child *must* be taught how to resolve
arguments without fighting, how to become street smart, and how
to avoid confrontations with violent peers. Parents *must* be cautious
about the potential for abuse by children and adults who provide
day-care, babysit, or visit the home.

If your child has epilepsy, be careful to prevent head injuries
during daily activities and seizures, but do not unnecessarily restrict
safe participation in the pursuits and challenges of childhood.
Suggestions about appropriate activities as the child ages are included in Chapters 16–19.

If a preventable accident caused your child's seizures, you can
become a powerful force for educating other parents about preventing head injuries. You can also help your child overcome any
resulting disability by promoting positive self-esteem and emphasizing what the child *can* do throughout life.

How Common Are Childhood Seizures?

Febrile seizures resulting from fever are the most common type
of childhood seizure, occurring in approximately one in thirty children. They indicate that a child has a somewhat lower threshold for
seizure activity, but do not necessarily mean that the child will
develop epilepsy. This is illustrated by the fact that over an entire
lifetime, one in eleven people (a little over 9 percent) will have a
seizure, whereas only three in one hundred people (3 percent) have
recurrent seizures that are diagnosed as epilepsy.

What Causes Seizures in Children?

The causes of seizures in children vary with age. Newborns are most susceptible to chemical imbalances and infections or brain damage in the uterus (see Chapter 12). Children between the ages of six months and four years are most likely to experience febrile seizures, but they may also have seizures from brain damage, infection, or metabolic problems. Breath-holding spells that look like seizures are most likely to occur in children between the ages of six months and four years.

What Should Be Done When a Child Has a Seizure?

Emergency medical help should be sought when a child has a first seizure. It is unlikely that the child's life is in danger, but it is best not to take chances because of the wide range of possible causes of seizures. The physician will usually want to see the child immediately. Medical personnel can gather information about the seizure that may help in making a diagnosis, and which the parents or others may have missed during the traumatic event.

Parents should learn about first aid (Chapter 11) after a child has had a seizure. Parents or others who are present when a child has a seizure need only make the child comfortable, remove any tight clothing, clear the area of dangerous objects, and talk soothingly to the child while the seizure takes its course. When the seizure is over, turn the child on his or her side to allow saliva or possible vomit to clear the mouth.

It is common for parents to fear that their child will die during a seizure, but that is very rare. Most childhood seizures last from a few seconds to a couple of minutes, and few involve the generalized tonic-clonic activity that can develop into status epilepticus (continuous epileptic activity), which can be life-threatening. If a child is at risk of status epilepticus, the parents should be instructed in the use of a rectal anticonvulsant.

What Kinds of Seizures Occur in Childhood and How Are They Treated?

Most children who develop epilepsy experience partial seizures. As described in Chapter 3, there are three types of partial seizures:

1. Simple partial seizures cause a single kind of movement or a strange sensation such as an emotion, smell, taste, or dizziness.

2. Complex partial seizures cause the child to lose awareness as the seizure begins, or the child loses awareness during a simple partial seizure. This is the most common type of epileptic seizure, affecting almost two-thirds of people with epilepsy.

3. A tonic-clonic seizure may occur following a partial seizure if it becomes generalized (affecting the whole body). A child having a tonic-clonic seizure may become rigid (tonic), fall to the ground, and begin shaking or jerking as the muscles relax and contract rhythmically (clonic).

Some children experience absence seizures (also called petit mal spells), in which they are unaware and unresponsive for a brief period. The child may stare or blink rapidly and is usually motionless and fails to respond when spoken to or touched. Absence seizures usually start between the ages of four and ten, and often cease as the child enters adulthood. Like febrile seizures, they tend to be inherited. Approximately half the children who have absence seizures also have at least one generalized tonic seizure.

Absence seizures can occur many times during the day, and they may go unnoticed by parents or teachers. They can cause sudden learning problems or behavioral changes. If a child continues to have frequent absence seizures, teachers and parents should help the child make up for missed information and remain socially connected to other children while treatment is maximized.

Several types of seizures may be triggered from different parts of the brain in children with severe brain damage. They may experience generalized seizures, in which there is an immediate loss of consciousness causing a fall, followed by clonic, tonic, or tonic-clonic seizure activity.

If various dosages and combinations of medications are unable to control seizures, surgery may be an option (see Chapter 10).

Patients rarely outgrow epilepsy, although children often outgrow absence seizures, but the age at which this occurs varies. However, not everyone with epilepsy has to take medication for their entire lifetime. As researchers learn more about the brain and the causes of epilepsy, the potential grows for more effective medications and surgeries—and possibly cures.

How Are Nonepileptic Seizures Treated?

Proper treatment of childhood seizures depends on prompt and thorough diagnostic testing to determine the cause (see Chapter 8). If a cause is found that can be corrected, such as a chemical imbalance, fever, or infection, treatment will most likely end the child's seizures. Otherwise, antiepileptic medications may be prescribed to help avoid repeated seizures. Although antiepileptic medications may be used, it is not correct to say the child has epilepsy if the underlying problem is thought to be correctable.

The most common cause of nonepileptic seizures in children is a high fever. Febrile seizures are usually of the generalized tonic-clonic type, especially between the ages of one and four years. This type of seizure tends to run in families, and it reflects an inherited seizure threshold that is lower than normal. Febrile seizures are seldom dangerous in themselves unless they last a long time or are repeated frequently. All febrile seizures should be evaluated by a physician to determine the cause of the fever and to decide if treatment with antiepileptic or other medications is necessary.

If the seizure is brief, the physician will probably treat the child with a cool bath and acetaminophen (Tylenol®). If the child has frequent febrile seizures, treatment with antiepileptic medications is usually initiated to raise the child's seizure threshold. The most commonly used medication is a small dose of phenobarbital. Phenobarbital is a safe and effective medication, but it can cause drowsiness in some children, slow learning in many, and hyperactivity in others. Other medications used for febrile seizures are valproic acid and carbamazepine. Fortunately, children usually outgrow febrile seizures as the brain matures, and treatment can be discontinued under a physician's supervision.

Some events are mistaken for seizures. For example, some children have breath-holding spells (also called apneic spells). They are most often seen in children between the ages of six months and four years and are usually provoked by pain, anger, or frustration. Although most tantrums and breath-holding spells do not cause seizures, a seizure can occur if the brain is temporarily deprived of oxygen.

A child experiencing breath-holding spells should be evaluated by a physician, even though they are seldom a sign of epilepsy. Parents can help a child overcome these spells by watching for signs of the cause of the behavior and by using behavior modification or other parenting skills discussed in Chapter 16. Be careful not to let the child associate this behavior with getting his own way, or breath-holding and seizure-like behavior may become a learned source of power over parents and other family members.

Another type of nonepileptic behavior is called a "psychogenic" seizure. Like a breath-holding spell, this behavior may mimic seizure activity but is not related to abnormal electrical activity in the brain. Psychogenic seizures are more common in adolescents and adults than in older children (see Chapter 15).

When Is It Necessary to See a Specialist?

All children with seizures should be evaluated by a pediatric neurologist promptly. This specialist can perform and interpret a series of EEG recordings to identify any underlying brain disorder that may be present. The pediatric neurologist can also help to reach a safe and effective medication dosage for the child's specific needs.

The child can then usually return to his or her pediatrician or family physician for routine care.

The child's primary physician should continue to consult with the pediatric neurologist about changes in medication or dosage. Medications can sometimes be discontinued after several months if no seizures occur and EEG recordings are normal, but this must be done very carefully under the direction of a pediatric neurologist.

If the child continues to experience seizures or has unacceptable side effects six months to a year after a first seizure, he should be evaluated at a specialized epilepsy center that has a wide range of health professionals who are experienced in dealing with seizures caused by epilepsy and by other physical or behavioral disorders. They can help the family deal with the entire range of challenges— physical, psychological, and social—that can be associated with childhood seizures.

When Should a Child Assume Responsibility for Taking Medications?

All children who must take any type of medication or other regular therapy can be participants in that process rather than being merely subjects of a parent's will. This is especially true of children with a disorder such as epilepsy (or diabetes), who may have to take medication for the rest of their lives. As the child matures, he can be given increasing responsibility for following the prescribed medication schedule. If scheduling problems or compliance difficulties occur, the child should be involved in the problem-solving process. The child's feelings of self-control and responsibility are nurtured by respect and trust.

A child as young as two years old can be involved in taking medications in very simple ways. Ask the child to help you find a convenient but "special" place to keep the medication. Let the child buy or choose a special spoon or cup to take the medication. Help him select or make stickers to put on a calendar as each dose is taken. Praise him, especially in front of others, for helping you remember the medication. If a dose is forgotten or is taken late, ask him to help you remember what the physician or nurse said to do. When you see the epilepsy care team, encourage the child's participation as much as possible. Never answer questions for a child who is capable of answering. Encourage him to express feelings and ask questions of health professionals.

As a child reaches school age, he can begin to assume responsibility for remembering to take medications. Include him in working with the physician to develop a schedule that does not require taking medications at school. If this cannot be avoided, you and your child should meet with the school nurse to work out a method that involves minimal interference with his classroom activities.

Include your child in discussions with teachers and other school officials about his epilepsy and what should be done if a seizure occurs. This should be handled in the spirit of helping everyone minimize the impact of the child's epilepsy, not seeking special attention or favors for him. Chapters 15 through 19 include more about coping in school and additional suggestions for helping a child assume greater responsibilities. The most important members of an infant's epilepsy team are the parents, who are fully responsible for their child's epilepsy care. As the child matures, he should gradually be given greater degrees of responsibility. By the time a child with epilepsy reaches adolescence, he will have become the most important member of the epilepsy team.

Your role as a parent is to help your child to successfully live with epilepsy. You cannot *make* this happen, but by encouraging your child to take responsibility for his health and happiness, you can increase the likelihood that he will be healthy and happy. By trusting your child to take risks and to learn from mistakes, you can increase the likelihood that your child will exceed everyone's expectations throughout life.

CHAPTER 15

TREATING SEIZURES IN ADOLESCENCE

From a medical point of view, treating seizures in adolescence is not very different from treating them in adults. You might wish to consult *Living Well with Epilepsy* (for patients and their families) or *The Epilepsy Handbook* (for physicians) for additional information.

The most common kind of seizures in adolescence are complex partial seizures. They begin in a small part of the brain and involve a disturbance of consciousness, although the patient may not completely lose all awareness or necessarily fall to the ground completely unconscious. The signs and symptoms of complex partial seizures are often subtle, and the diagnosis is often missed or delayed. Consciousness is quickly restored after an absence seizure. After a complex partial seizure, even a brief one, the child may be slightly confused or not quite "with it" for several minutes; she may have a headache or feel a need to sleep. Many antiepileptic medications are effective in treating complex partial seizures, and they are also most likely to be successfully treated with surgery.

Absence seizures are normally seen in children between the ages of four and twelve years, but they may persist into adolescence. If so, they are often more difficult to treat. It is important that your physician be able to distinguish absence seizures of the classic type or those associated with juvenile myoclonic epilepsy from those atypical absence seizures caused by diffuse brain damage. Absence seizures have a typical 3 per second spike wave appearance on the EEG in which the activity is bilateral—it appears at the same moment on both sides of the head and in equal amplitude. They are often provoked by hyperventilation. Atypical absence seizures often have a much slower rate of discharge, about 2 to 2 1/2 times per second, have less well-ordered EEG, may be associated with tonic seizures, and are usually found in children who have brain damage.

One particular kind of seizure that has a strong hereditary component and appears particularly in adolescence is juvenile myoclonic epilepsy, or Janz syndrome. The hallmark of these seizures is that the adolescent often suddenly throws an arm about, especially early in the morning. A common story is that "my child tosses the hairbrush in the bathroom when she wakes up." Juvenile myoclonic epilepsy may also be associated with prolonged absence or generalized tonic-clonic seizures. It tends to disappear in young adulthood and can often be well-controlled with standard antiepileptic drugs, particularly valproic acid. The EEG may resemble that seen with absence seizures.

Adolescence is a stormy time from a psychological and social point of view. Most parents find raising adolescents to be a challenge. With the added complication of epilepsy and antiepileptic drugs, both parent and child often need outside counseling. In my experience, three issues tend to surface repeatedly: disturbances in mood, problems with compliance, and difficulty in developing a positive self-image and a strong ego. Whether or not a child has epilepsy, a teenager who is moody, withdrawn, and irritable, and who acts out in other ways, may be depressed or otherwise in need of psychological counseling. The earlier the teenager has a chance to express frustration and anger and comes to grips with the unique challenges that life has presented the better.

Western society places a high premium on always being in control and doing the right thing. When a seizure occurs, the child is not in control and does not always do the right thing. (How do you answer your teacher promptly and politely if you are in the middle of a seizure or somewhat confused postictally?). Antiepileptic medications may cause difficulty in concentration or learning. If this is not recognized and dealt with, a child may not do as well in school as parents, teachers, or the child expect. These factors and many others lead to poor self-image and a sense of failure, or at least a sense of being different. Warm parental support and understanding are necessary and may be all that is needed.

However, this is the kind of a problem that creates major difficulties throughout life if it not dealt with early and promptly. Nothing leads to a sense of failure and lack of self-worth more than repeated failures and rebuffs. Ask your physician, school counselor, or local social agency for help if your child shows these kinds of symptoms. It is rather natural and not uncommon for a child to be angry because she is sick. That is a perfectly normal human response. It is also a normal human response to displace that anger onto someone else, especially someone we love and admire.

Low blood levels of antiepileptic medication do not always indicate noncompliance. Children grow rapidly during adolescence and hormonal changes occur as the child goes through puberty. These changes, as well as other medications the child may be taking, affect the metabolism of antiepileptic drugs. As a result, frequent dosage adjustments may be necessary.

Talk of suicide or a desire to hurt oneself or hurt someone else should never be ignored or dismissed. Suicide and depression are common in adolescence, and having uncontrolled seizures and difficulty adjusting to the disorder is a frequent precipitator of depression. This kind of talk is a sign that the child is reaching out for help. The child often talks to friends rather than directly to her parents. The child usually cannot express the frustration and desperation that she feels. Unfortunately, most of us feel threatened and anxious if a child talks about depression or suicide and we try to brush it off. This is one instance in which we need to be strong and seek professional help.

Alcohol, Caffeine, and Recreational Drugs

The interaction between various medications and drugs is complex. Antiepileptic medications are particularly prone to interaction with other chemicals. The consumption of alcohol, tobacco, caffeine, and street drugs can affect the metabolism of antiepileptic medications.

Alcohol

A few people find that alcohol makes their seizures worse. Most people taking antiepileptic medications report that they have a lower tolerance for alcohol and that they quickly become high or drunk. This is particularly dangerous for adolescents, who are probably unaccustomed to drinking. Teenagers should experiment with the effects of alcohol in the safety of their home so that they can be more responsible when they are out with their friends. Antiepileptic medications and driving are a problem—and mixing antiepileptic medications, drinking, and driving is a *very serious* problem. Remember that falls and pedestrian accidents can easily occur if someone is drunk. Not everyone recognizes that drinking contests often involve fatally toxic amounts of alcohol before the person becomes too drunk to continue.

Alcohol increases the metabolism of many AEDs and may require larger doses.

Caffeine

Caffeine is prevalent in American society. We find it in coffee, cola drinks (there are particularly large amounts in Jolt and Mountain Dew), tea, and chocolate. Most people taking antiepileptic medications can consume moderate amounts of caffeine without difficulty. A rule of thumb is that three cups of coffee or three soft drinks a day do not cause trouble. However, drinking five, ten, or fifteen cups of coffee a day, as many people do, often lowers the seizure threshold.

Smoking

Nicotine increases the metabolism of many antiepileptic drugs and creates the need for higher doses. Alcohol does the same. In general, smoking is dangerous to one's health, and the combination of smoking, drinking, and antiepileptic medications makes it very difficult for the physician to arrive at a proper dosage.

Street or Recreational Drugs

These drugs are dangerous, particularly to those with epilepsy. One of the biggest problems is that you never know what you are buying. In fact, one can assume that LSD, speed (amphetamines), heroin, cocaine, or marijuana obtained on the street is adulterated (not pure). The chemicals that are mixed in often make seizures worse or interfere with antiepileptic medications.

Some patients have told me that marijuana helps their seizures, and there have been a number of newspaper reports discussing marijuana and seizures. Marijuana certainly is not a strong antiepileptic drug. I am unconvinced that marijuana is useful in the treatment of epilepsy. On the other hand, I have not seen any evidence that moderate amounts of marijuana used recreationally make seizures worse.

Exercise and Athletics

Exercise and athletics are particularly important for adolescents, a period in which we build our body and develop general body strength and bone density. Exercise rarely causes a problem with seizures, but the psychological stress of competitive athletics sometimes does. Most people with epilepsy find that regular, strenuous exercise is helpful.

What we need to watch out for is the *kind* of athletic activity. People with seizures who are likely to lose consciousness must take certain precautions. They must not engage in athletic events in which the loss of consciousness can cause injury to the patient or others. This includes automobile racing, flying an airplane, sky diving, scuba diving, technical rock climbing and mountain climbing, working on the high bar and the high rings, and heavy contact sports such as football, lacrosse, and rugby.

Sports such as soccer, basketball, baseball, track and field, field hockey, ice hockey, archery, tennis, badminton, squash, racquetball, and others may be strongly encouraged.

Three common sports need to be discussed in detail.

Bicycle riding. Bicycle riding in the city or on roads with heavy traffic is dangerous for anyone. If a child has frequent seizures, bicycle riding may be a problem. However, ordinary bicycle riding for anyone whose seizures are not severely uncontrolled is usually safe as long as a helmet is worn.

Swimming. The most common form of accidental death for people with epilepsy is drowning. However, they are just as likely to drown in three inches of water in the bathtub as they are swimming. Swimming in clear water with a buddy immediately at hand and ready assistance is permissible for all but people with the most severe cases of epilepsy. It is good exercise. However, it requires constant vigilance, and people with epilepsy have drowned in indoor swimming pools under the eyes of lifeguards because the lifeguard's attention was distracted by an event elsewhere and there was nobody immediately next to the swimmer.

Horseback riding. Horseback riding is one of the most dangerous sports if measured by the frequency of head injury. People whose seizures are well-controlled are at no greater risk while riding than anyone else. However, those who have seizures as frequently as once a month would be well advised not to ride a horse. Of course, if a gentle horse is being led by an experienced adult or special precautions for handicapped children are being taken, the activity is usually safe.

CHAPTER 16

LIVING WELL WITH EPILEPSY: THE PRESCHOOL YEARS

This chapter is not intended to be a substitute for the many books that provide advice on being a good parent. Rather, it concentrates on some of the specific issues that arise from having epilepsy.

When a child is diagnosed with epilepsy (or any other chronic disorder), there is a natural tendency for parents to feel guilty—to believe that they somehow failed to protect their child and that the illness is their fault. This is rarely the case, and a parent's inappropriate sense of guilt may worsen the situation. Parents should seek counseling if this type of guilt is weighing heavily on them. We almost never know the cause of epilepsy, and only rarely is a child involved in an avoidable accident that could somehow be blamed on the parent. Even those cases of epilepsy that are related to a strong genetic component should not be a source of guilt for the parent, who probably did not know anything about the problem at the time the child was conceived.

By definition, life is risky and always ends in death. A reasonable risk of accidents must be accepted or a child would not be able to explore the world and grow up to become a functioning adult. It is a natural and normal parental desire to protect our children, but we must not allow that desire to lead us to smother the child. Rather, parents must resolve to do everything possible to help the child overcome the challenges of epilepsy and to live well.

Learning to live well with epilepsy for a child is like learning to use the body and learning to exercise. It takes patience and practice before the child increases his skills. Epilepsy is less frightening to the parents and the child when they understand it. Many of the families I have treated have developed entirely new ways of coping with difficult problems by accepting the fact that it is a gradual process that must be practiced. I hope you and your family can use this book to reach and grow.

If there is any lesson I wish I had learned when I raised my own children, it is that when a parent gets excited and overreacts, the child gets excited and overreacts. A major step in helping your child become a calm and resourceful adult is to modulate your reaction to the seriousness of the situation. Ignoring minor issues, distracting the child engaged in somewhat more risky behavior, and making a big issue only when a situation is truly dangerous (running across the street in front of a car, for example) are good rules for raising any child.

Many parents cannot control their adrenaline rush and excitement and overreact. Some become so anxious that they lose their temper and spank or shake the child inappropriately, while others just feel helpless and give up any sense of trying to direct the child. If you recognize yourself in these words, then you, the parent, should seek help early so that you will be able to help your child appropriately.

Some Common Mistakes in Raising a Child with Epilepsy

If we make a big fuss about things, the child picks up on that and often places grave importance on things that are irrelevant. Treat going to the physician or taking medication matter of factly. A parent can take a vitamin pill or a glass of fruit juice when the child takes his pills as a way of just making this seem like an ordinary family activity. If your child turns this into a contest of wills, seek professional advice as soon as possible. That will make for a much easier time, especially as the child enters adolescence.

It is impossible not to be upset to some extent when a child has a seizure. Children often interpret this as displeasure with their behavior. Hug and support your child and love him rather than get upset over wet underwear or fuss about something irrelevant.

Don't make too much of a fuss about each seizure or that behavior may turn seizures into an attention-getting device. The last thing we want to do is give the child a present or so much attention after each seizure that he begins to fake seizures to get attention.

Epilepsy is not an excuse for misbehavior, nor should the child with epilepsy be treated more favorably than his brothers and sisters. That only creates resentment in the family or a sense of undeserved entitlement in the child.

Unfortunately, some families still think that there is something wrong or "dirty" about having seizures. If you never discuss the child's epilepsy or whisper about it as if it is something secret or frightening, the child will get all the wrong signals. The child and his brothers and sisters will become fearful and he will have difficulty developing a strong positive ego.

Keep epilepsy and seizures in perspective, and be prepared to run some risks. Help your child learn to grow normally and work around the epilepsy, rather that focusing on it as a problem.

That is why early diagnosis and intervention are so important. We can help our children see themselves as healthy, growing, learning people, in whom epilepsy is just one more thing to be considered along with the walk to school and whether or not we can drink milk. (For example, many Blacks, Asians, American Indians, and people from the Mediterranean area are lactose intolerant and their children cannot drink milk.) This attitude helps the child grow normally. I wish that every child who had seizures could have them under complete control before they go to school. In my experience, those children grow up to be completely normal adults. Simply because seizures are less physically dangerous to a preschool child than they are to an adult is not a reason to ignore them or to wait and see what happens. Children rarely outgrow epilepsy (except for some with classic absence seizures). If your physician does not take your child's seizures seriously, if he does not do everything possible to stop them completely, you should seek expert help from a specialized epilepsy center.

We used to worry about how a child related to his peers when beginning school. With more mothers working, many children go to day-care and preschool. How other children, and even more importantly, teachers and the parents of other children, view the child with epilepsy and respond to his seizure becomes very important. This subject is discussed in the next chapter on the elementary school years.

CHAPTER 17

LIVING WELL WITH EPILEPSY— THE ELEMENTARY SCHOOL YEARS

In general, children up to the age of two or three do not seem to measure themselves against each other and tend to play more or less alone. But by the time a child is involved in preschool and neighborhood playing, and certainly by the time he or she enters kindergarten, the measuring process begins. The child observes other children—how they behave, how they look—and how other children and adults respond to them. The child experiences acceptance and rejection, support and discipline. Competition begins, whether in a foot race or in grading of school work. In other words, peer pressure from outside the family becomes important in creating behavior patterns.

These factors are important for how *all* children develop a feeling of self-esteem. A child who has had strong support and adequate reward at home enters into the world with an advantage over one who has been neglected or put down.

However, the presence of epilepsy introduces complications. Unless other children, teachers, and parents understand that seizures are an uncontrolled behavior, the child can easily become looked upon as different or strange and be ridiculed when a seizure occurs at school. Children are very sensitive to the feelings of others; they become embarrassed and develop a sense of negative self-worth as the result of experiencing seizures in front of others. Yet we cannot protect children from this or they will not grow up to become functioning adults. Helping your child steer a safe course through these conflicting obstacles is the main subject of this chapter.

A child's self-image and self-esteem are largely determined by parental comments and actions. The parents' role is so important that it is often impossible for a teacher, another adult, or even a skilled therapist to undo damage to a child's self-esteem created in the early years of life by the parent. Similarly, if a parent has taken the time to build a child's self-esteem and self-confidence, it will help that child throughout life against negative, thoughtless, or cruel comments from other adults or children. Remember, however, that no parent is in complete control and many good and bad things shape our children no matter how hard we try.

We need to steer a course between extremes. Paying a great deal of supervisory attention to a child, but only to scold, caution, or protect, will help that child grow up to think that she is in need of close supervision or protection. If a child is mostly ignored and left to fend for herself, she may well think of herself as not deserving attention and will have difficulty forming close relationships later in life. Many excellent books discuss such general factors in great detail.

A problem can occur if a child with epilepsy is treated as deserving special attention. Especially if epilepsy is used as an excuse at home, it may become an excuse for all types of misbehavior and avoidance of responsibility. This may set in motion a damaging cycle of relationships. The child may use epilepsy as an excuse to not pay attention or to withdraw from interactions with other children. Any attempt by the teacher or other adults to help the child may result in denial or angry attempts by the parents to protect the child, thus reinforcing the child's behavior. Pretty soon everyone is angry with everyone else.

If the school reports a problem, thank the teacher for contacting you and then try to understand what the issues are and to work them out. Most teachers are very understanding and supportive. Some may need additional information about epilepsy (which they can obtain by reading this book and by contacting your local chapter of the Epilepsy Foundation of America). Others may have unfortunate attitudes, in which case it may be necessary to involve other school authorities as you work out a suitable action plan for your child at school.

Most children with epilepsy do not require special treatment at school. But if a child must take medication during the day or avoid certain types of activities, be sure to discuss it with the teacher and the school nurse and involve your physician in planning if necessary.

Medication Issues

Taking medication during the day can often be avoided by administering it just before the child goes to school and when she comes back in mid-afternoon. This avoids many difficulties since many schools are very concerned about children taking pills and confuse the need for medication with the problems of street drugs.

Having a seizure at school often creates an unnecessary amount of excitement. Again, prior planning and discussion go a long way toward heading off problems. If your child has frequent seizures, explain to the teacher what might happen and how to provide the necessary first aid. In that way you can avoid having to run to the school each time there is a seizure (or even worse, have the child sent home every time one occurs).

In general, if the child has a seizure that is typical and self-limited and does not present new problems, it is best to let her recover and return to class. Of course, that may not be possible if the child's typical seizure is a major generalized tonic-clonic seizure and she faces two or three hours of postictal sleep.

Helping the teacher learn to observe the seizure and giving her the information she needs to feel that some degree of control over the situation will go a long way toward minimizing the social and emotional impact of having a seizure at school. On the other hand, work with your physician to provide your teacher with clear, good guidelines about when a seizure is an emergency and when to have the child taken immediately to an emergency room. Above all, work together so that the child does not decide that seizures are a good way to get out of class and avoid going to school.

Making Friends

Children with epilepsy need not have a more difficult time making friends than anyone else. They will have no problems if they have a reasonably good self-image. Help build your child's confidence and self-esteem at home so that she can develop more confidence in social situations.

The best way to help your child make friends is to encourage desirable social behavior and to praise her when she behaves appropriately. Nothing special need be done simply because the child has epilepsy.

How Do I Explain My Child's Epilepsy to Others?

It is always easier if you have a good relationship with the people with whom you want to discuss your child's epilepsy. Try to meet neighbors and parents of neighborhood children. Discuss your mutual interests and those of your child. See if it makes sense for your children to play together. Epilepsy will enter into the discussion depending upon how likely it is that your child may have a seizure while playing. Try to avoid surprises. Don't try to hide the fact that your child has epilepsy and do try to provide enough mation to the other parents so that they will respond appropriately if your child has a seizure in their home. This book, as well as pamphlets available from the Epilepsy Foundation of America, will provide basic facts about epilepsy so that the other parents have no misconceptions. Give them simple first-aid tips and reassure them that they don't need to do anything to treat the seizure. Let them know how and when to call for help. Thank them for understanding and for helping your child to have a chance to develop socially.

It is often helpful to include your child when you tell others about epilepsy. Ask her how she would like it explained. Help the child learn to introduce the subject in an appropriate manner and at appropriate times—after a friend has gotten to know something about her as an individual.

It is particularly important that as the child gets older you let her assume greater responsibility for introducing the subject and explaining epilepsy. This will provide a valuable skill when meeting people throughout life.

Day-Care and Babysitters

All parents needs an occasional break from children, to be alone both as individuals and as a couple. Children also benefit from these breaks because they learn to survive even when mom and dad aren't there (see Chapters 23 and 24).

Summer Camp

Summer camp is a wonderful opportunity for children. Children with epilepsy should have the opportunity to go. The child whose seizures are very well controlled may be able to go to a normal camp. The child with occasional seizures or even with seizures that are difficult to control may benefit from a special camp for children with epilepsy.

Just as with day-care, visit the camp and talk to the staff ahead of time. Of course, if the camp is one for children with epilepsy, the staff will already be well-trained and all you will need to do is give them specifics about your child.

The camp experience is an important step in building self-esteem and confidence. It is a wonderful opportunity for more socialization and in gaining self-reliance. And of course, the more confident and self-reliant a child is, the easier it is to let her participate more fully in life when you are not around.

Special Help at School

Public Law 94-192, the "Education for All Handicapped Children Act," requires that all public school districts give an adequate education to children regardless of handicaps. The law requires that a handicapped child participate in regular classrooms as long as she is able to benefit from the experience more than from attending a specially adapted program. Most children with epilepsy can participate fully in regular classrooms.

Most schools try to do whatever they can to help any child with a handicap. Parents of children with epilepsy should meet with the child's teacher at least once a year, and with the administrators and school nurse as necessary, to discuss their perceptions of how your child is doing and your own particular concerns.

Should I Tell the School That My Child Has Epilepsy If the Seizures Are Well-Controlled?

In general, I believe the answer is yes. Should an unexpected seizure occur, the school will be forewarned and it will not be a major crisis. Furthermore, specific advantages are afforded a child under the Education for All Handicapped Children Act, of which you may wish to take advantage. It is especially important to openly discuss with school personnel any other kind of brain damage, difficulty in learning, or difficulty in socialization that your child may have.

For your child to receive the most from school, it is important that the teacher feel comfortable about epilepsy in general and be informed about your child. A letter from your physician and specific instructions from you will be particularly helpful. Take advantage of the Epilepsy Foundation's programs to instruct teachers in first aid for seizures.

Parents can also suggest that the teacher discuss epilepsy with the child's classmates. Programs for doing this are available from the Epilepsy Foundation and from the MINCEP® Epilepsy Program at Gillette Children's Hospital in St. Paul, Minnesota. Your child can be involved in doing a presentation in class. Epilepsy can be placed in context with other disorders that affect children such as diabetes.

The most embarrassing thing that can happen to a child is to have a seizure involving convulsions and loss of urinary or bowel control in front of a large group of children. Recovery from this experience depends largely on how the teacher handles the incident and discusses it with classmates. Parents can help by suggesting appropriate ways for a teacher to explain epilepsy to different age groups.

For example, preschoolers tend to be very open about asking questions about what they have observed. Most of all, the teacher needs to reassure them that the child who had the seizure will be fine. The teacher can distract them by giving them something else to do while the child is cared for. Afterwards the teacher can explain that Tommy's brain told him to have a seizure but that he is okay now. They should be told that they are not going to have a seizure, they can't "catch" it from Tommy, and that neither they nor Tommy did anything to cause it. They should know that the child may have another seizure some other time, but they can play with him just like before and needn't worry. The important thing with preschoolers is to dispel fear.

Elementary school teachers can use slides, movies, and classroom instruction to provide education about epilepsy. Children in this age range are most concerned about safety for themselves and their classmates. They want to know if Tommy can control when a seizure occurs. They also need to be reassured that they won't develop the disorder. The main objective with this age group is to provide accurate information and to prevent the development of false ideas or ridicule as a result of having a seizure at school.

In high school the approach can become much more intellectual. Students understand specific teaching about epilepsy. They are better able to generalize from their classmate's seizure to a health disorder affecting large numbers of people. Seizures can be discussed in the context of how the brain functions and how electrical activity in the brain can develop an abnormal pattern that causes a seizure. High school students usually focus less on safety and more on what they can do to help. It may be particularly effective for the student with epilepsy to do a written or oral report on epilepsy and to lead the class discussion on chronic health disorders. It is important that high school teachers build a positive attitude among classmates so that if a seizure does occur they are more likely to want to do something to help their classmate rather than to ridicule him or to run away.

Of course, there will always be some children and adults who bully or ridicule others. The child with epilepsy and his classmates need to understand that they cannot control such people. They *can* control how they feel about themselves and about each other. We need to help our child to understand that these comments reflect the person making them, rather than internalizing the comments as true reflections of their own qualities. If the child with epilepsy is confident and asserts that people who ridicule others are the ones with the real problem, peers and teachers will admire his strength of character. With epilepsy, you benefit most when the school, teachers, and students create an attitude of acceptance and understanding. This is becoming much more difficult to obtain. Larger cities and schools suffer from cultural violence, and preying on the weak has become a way of life.

CHAPTER 18

LIVING WELL WITH EPILEPSY— ADOLESCENCE

Please have your teenager read this chapter, perhaps even with you.

Of all of the ages of man, adolescence is a time of extremes. We seem to feel our emotions particularly keenly at that time: happiness and sadness, love and hate, excitement and anger. Some of us thrive on the stormy feelings, others find them painful. Adolescence is seldom an easy time either for teenagers or for those close to them. It is a time when young people feel the need to make decisions and act independently. It is hard enough for parents of children without epilepsy to accept this and take risks; it is particularly difficult if you are worried about your child's health and safety.

Whether you have epilepsy or not, one factor that helps contribute to a positive experience during adolescence is the ability and the feeling of freedom to communicate. Not enforced family conferences, but an atmosphere in which both child and parent can openly discuss their concerns with each other and with friends. In an atmosphere of mutual concern and support, boundaries can be set for both the teenager and parents through mutual discussion about the reasons for limitations.

Adolescence is a crucial time for someone with epilepsy. All adolescents are busy developing a self-concept and coping abilities to live in the world—a world designed primarily for people without health problems. Epilepsy is an additional stressor in this transition. The teenager with epilepsy does not look different from his friends, but may be acutely aware of the difference and may exaggerate it in his internal emotions. As an added problem, the teenager with epilepsy may not be allowed to do some of the things that his peers are doing. This chapter discusses some of the issues that impact on all teenagers, focusing particularly on epilepsy and its special needs.

It is not always a good idea to keep epilepsy a secret from others. At one time, secrecy regarding epilepsy was very common because of public fear and official discrimination against those with epilepsy. This has changed. Although there is still too much public misunderstanding, families, epilepsy organizations, and physicians have been able to make a big difference in how the world views people with epilepsy. The biggest problem is that not enough people are willing to talk openly about epilepsy and to educate others.

The big problem with secrecy is that it helps create a negative self-image. If you keep something secret, you must be ashamed of it, right? And most of us are not very good at keeping secrets or telling lies. What an added strain to carry this burden! Too often, trying to keep epilepsy a secret leads to social withdrawal and isolation, which create major problems in how we live our lives. A better approach is to look at epilepsy as just another way in which people can be different. It is a nuisance to have seizures, but three out of every one hundred people have them. Most of these people have overcome having seizures to lead active, happy lives.

The decision about who and when and how to tell about epilepsy should be made by the child and parents together.

Teachers, coaches, and other school officials should definitely be informed, and the family should meet with them to discuss how medications and seizures should be handled. Perhaps you won't have any difficulty from your medications and it doesn't really matter all that much. Others will have good days and bad days, and teachers need to know what to expect.

You should tell those friends with whom you spend a great deal of time because they need to know what kind of seizures you have and what to do in case one occurs. These friends should also know whether you want them to tell others that you have epilepsy. Remember that a lot of how you handle your epilepsy is determined by how frequent and how serious your seizures are. If seizures rarely or never occur during the day, you may choose to tell only your closest friends. This prevents others from judging you based on prior beliefs about epilepsy. Your friends need to know they have nothing to fear but that they can offer much in the way of understanding and support. This sharing of personal information will increase the bond between you and your friends. If you have frequent seizures at school, you must be open about discussing epilepsy in classes and with everyone who asks. This will not only help dispel misunderstandings, but also may reduce the tendency of teenagers to ridicule and humiliate those who are different. Most teenagers feel empathy for and want to be helpful to those who are dealing with a chronic health disorder. They will admire you if you handle your epilepsy confidently and without fear.

Some people will make fun of you, be mean to you, or be afraid of you, just as they would with anyone who is visibly different. You can do little about their behavior. Just realize that they are not the type of people you want to be your friends. The best way to discourage their mean behavior is to try not to be visibly upset by it so that they don't obtain any gratification. If others see that a bully's teasing has little effect or backfires, they will side with the person being teased. This further discourages the bully. Laughing at the bully and making the bully an object of ridicule is a very good defense.

If the actions of a bully become violent, a teenager needs to feel confident that school officials will be helpful. This can be a particular problem in the 1990s as violence invades our schools. If you have doubt about being able to rely on school officials, you and your parents should meet with them and decide how to prevent further problems.

Epilepsy Need Not Keep You from Leading a Normal Life

Epilepsy does not necessarily affect a teenager's ability to lead a normal life and become an independent adult, but it does tend to confuse matters. Adolescents face many challenges as they enter puberty, begin dating, experience the stresses of high school, and make decisions about how to make a living. All teenagers find themselves bewildered at times. It is hard to ride the hormonal and psychological roller coaster of adolescence. Epilepsy only adds another confusing factor.

The family's response to epilepsy during preschool and school years and how they handle the added stresses of the teen years will greatly influence the teenager's self-image and self-esteem. If a pattern of open communication and positive reinforcement has been established, the family will more likely weather any crises that occur. Open communication is the best defense against the risks that cut off a teenager's receptiveness to parental love and guidance.

Parents who have the healthiest relationships with their teenagers tend to be those who feel it is their responsibility to help the child mature into an independent adult. Parents whose children have the most trouble becoming independent seem to be those who feel that their major responsibility is to protect the child from harm. We need to set realistic limits to protect our children but must accept the fact that every child encounters risks in life. To protect our children from every risk denies them the ability to learn to face the world independently.

How to Deal with Rebellious Behavior

Most teens will argue with or disobey a parent at some time, no matter what type of relationship has developed over the years. Part of becoming independent is to have ideas of your own, to want to make your own decisions about your behavior, and to test these ideas. However, there may be times of open rebellion, which can be the toughest test of a parent's patience and love. This is when an adolescent most needs the parents' help and support. It is easy and common for a health disorder such as diabetes or epilepsy to become the focus of rebellion. Many people deny that they have an illness or insist that it will go away soon. They refuse to take medications or deliberately do things that cause a seizure. Parents can assist by gently helping these teens see the consequences of skipping medication. If a seizure occurs because medications were missed, don't dwell on the seizure or on the fact that it could have been prevented. Rather, focus on the future, expressing confidence that the teenager will want to be as healthy and active as possible and will want to take medications to avoid the seizures. Find a way to remember to take medications, to get enough rest, and to eat properly without nagging about it. Help the teenager understand that these are his own responsibilities. Remind the teenager that the reward for these actions is feeling good, not having seizures, and, most importantly, being able to do the things that really matter in his life, such as driving a car!

Drugs and Medication

One of the most important decisions a teenager must make is whether or not to go along with peers and break the law by drinking alcohol or taking illegal drugs. There is no doubt of the potential damage that alcohol and drugs can cause, but there is also no denying the fact that some people have survived repeated drunken or drug-induced experiences without becoming addicted or suffering other consequences. Each person must consider what they want to achieve in life and whether it is worth risking the physical, emotional, and social dangers involved with the illegal use of drugs and alcohol.

Serious risks exist even if the street drug that you take is exactly what you have been told it is. Most drugs affect the brain—that's how they work, but that's also where seizures originate. Therefore, the effect of a drug on people with epilepsy is likely to be a double whammy, often increasing the chance of a seizure. Illegal drugs, especially uppers and downers, can be very dangerous when mixed with antiepileptic medications.

Epilepsy and Dating

I am the last person to claim to be an expert on teenage dating, but here are some of the things my patients have taught me.

Everyone is nervous when they begin dating or when they begin dating a new person. There is no reason to make yourself more nervous by talking about epilepsy before you are comfortable doing so. It may be better to first date someone who already knows you have epilepsy. If that is impossible, decide whether your date needs to know about your epilepsy for safety reasons. If not, wait until you are comfortable with each other and then bring up the subject the same way you did with your friends of the same sex.

When first dating, arrange a group date. This makes conversation easier and helps everyone get to know each other without the pressure of being alone.

Before asking someone for a date or when trying to attract someone's interest, try to get to know them better at school or the group where you met them. Talk with him or her in class or wherever else you have the opportunity. After a few conversations, his or her reaction will give you a good idea about whether or not he is willing to date you. Find out what the other person likes to do and suggest it as something you could do together. That works as well for girls as for boys. Many boys are too shy to ask a girl out even if they like her. But if a girl is friendly and begins to discuss an activity, the boy may be encouraged to ask her out, or she can ask him out.

Don't give up if you are turned down when you ask for a date. Your friend may just want to get to know you better before dating or may be too shy. If he or she avoids you, turn your attention to someone else. Everyone experiences rejection at some time in their life. If you continue to be friendly, you will find that there is always someone who wants to get to know you better.

If you have trouble making conversation, arrange to do something active on the first date. Bowling or an outdoor activity may be better than going out to eat where you will be alone with the other person and feel more pressure to think of things to talk about.

Remember that dating should be enjoyable. Don't put so much pressure on yourself that you turn it into a tense, exhausting experience. That is likely to happen if you worry too much about how to impress the other person or whether or not to kiss or make out. For some reason, one of the hardest things to do when first dating someone is to act yourself. The more you relax and let things happen naturally, the more you will enjoy dating.

It is natural to want to engage in kissing and other intimate sharing. Let these things come gradually, as you become more comfortable with each other. Talk about your feelings and find out what the other person is comfortable with before you try to become more intimate.

CHAPTER 19

LIVING WELL WITH EPILEPSY— THE YOUNG ADULT

There is far more to be said here than can be handled in a single chapter. For this reason, I have written a separate book called *Living Well with Epilepsy* (New York: Demos Vermande, 1996). Any adult with epilepsy will find this book useful.

The ultimate role of a parent is to help a child mature and learn to live independently. Many factors influence a parent's ability to fulfill this role. For the parent of an adult child with epilepsy, the most important factor is the severity of the child's seizure disorder. Almost all children with epilepsy grow up to be independent adults. However, a few individuals with severe epilepsy may need to live in group homes or with some type of supervised care, either from parents or from health professionals. This is rarely because of seizures alone, but because the brain damage that caused the seizure leads to the necessity for special care. Perhaps even more common than brain damage as a cause for needing to live in a group home are serious psychological disturbances which would require that the young adult live in a structured and protected environment whether or not they had seizures (see Chapter 24).

No matter how an adult child is affected by epilepsy, parents can help their child overcome challenges and reach goals. These may include getting a job, going to college, moving out of the parents' home, or becoming involved in social activities.

Professional Assessment of Abilities

Disagreement and conflict about independence sometimes arise between an older teen or adult with epilepsy and her parents. One side feels that the person with epilepsy is capable of more independence, while the other does not think independence is a realistic goal. Sometimes parents disagree with each other about this issue, sometimes both parents encourage more independence than the adult child is willing to attempt, and sometimes the adult child pushes for more independence than parents think is reasonable or safe.

Because of the emotional involvement of each of the parties in these disputes, it is often helpful to obtain professional advice. The best person to do this is a family counselor who is familiar with epilepsy and with the services available to help people with disabilities live independently or in group homes. The counselor listens to each person's viewpoint, consults with the epilepsy team and the person with epilepsy about her abilities and desires, and then presents reasonable options for the family to discuss and consider. The counselor can also advise the family about community resources for people with disabilities, such as job training programs and assisted living arrangements.

With a professional assessment of the adult child's abilities, the family can set reasonable goals and begin to work toward them. The following are suggestions to increase the chances of achieving goals:

> ✥ For each goal, write a plan that includes the steps that need to be taken in order to reach the goal. For each step, decide on several actions that the person with epilepsy must do (perhaps with help from others) to reach the next step.

For example, if the goal is to get a job, the first step is to assess what type of jobs the person is capable of doing. A few occupations are not open to people with epilepsy, including some jobs in public transportation (pilot, train engineer, bus driver, interstate truck driver) and the military (although certain noncombat positions are open to people with epilepsy, and combat positions are open to those who have been off medications and seizure-free for at least five years). The next step is to choose an occupation or job in which the person is interested. After learning what qualifications are required, a series of steps could lead the person through the process of acquiring those qualifications and then applying for positions. Chapter 22 includes more information about careers and applying for jobs.

✧ After a realistic plan is written, everyone in the family can help by being supportive and positive about the person's abilities and efforts. There is no place for negative or skeptical comments, especially when the person is having difficulty achieving a step. Congratulate and reward good effort as well as actual achievements.

✧ If, after the best efforts of the person with epilepsy, it appears that a goal is not achievable, help the person avoid feelings of personal inadequacy that lower self-esteem. Go back to the plan and decide if some steps can be changed or broken into smaller, more achievable steps. Perhaps the goal needs to be changed. The important thing is to help the person stay motivated and keep trying to achieve important goals.

What Is the Best Living Arrangement?

Every family goes through a process of deciding how best to help a child attain a happy and active life. A major part of this decision process is weighing the benefits and drawbacks of various living arrangements. A wide range of alternatives exist, each with positive and negative aspects. Options must be weighed according to each child's personality, abilities, and desires, with recognition of the parents' circumstances and desires and in the light of financial realities. Decisions should not be based on arbitrary rules or practices established by custom, parents, or others (for example, some families who feel that once a child reaches an arbitrary age such as eighteen or twenty-one, she must leave home and "make it on her own" without parental assistance).

Seizure control is likely to play a major factor in determining an adult child's ability to live independently. The fact that a child continues to have seizures should not be used as a reason to rule out independent living. First, consider whether everything possible has been done to prevent seizures and undesirable side effects. Improved epilepsy control may lead to employment and enhanced self-confidence, which will make the adult child and parents more comfortable with an independent living arrangement. A consultation at an epilepsy center with comprehensive psychological and social resources should be considered.

If an adult child continues to have seizures, consider whether they truly require a parent's supervision or interfere with the person's ability to live away from home. It may be possible to find a suitable roommate or hire an aide to give the child a chance at independent living. Try to give the young adult a chance to succeed. Find appropriate help and do not react negatively to the challenges that all young people face when they live away from home for the first time (such as lax housekeeping standards). Parents can continue to help with financial and practical matters, but they should respect boundaries set by the child, such as only visiting when invited.

Another possibility for an adult child whose seizures prevent completely independent living may be a group home for people with epilepsy and similar disorders. These homes are supervised by trained counselors or other health professionals, and they are often financed by state or federal programs. They can offer adults with disabilities a chance to socialize with others and to engage in activities that they might otherwise be unable to pursue. Unfortunately, the quality of the facilities and supervision can range from very good to very bad. Seek references from your epilepsy team or the local affiliate of the Epilepsy Foundation of America. Then take your son or daughter to visit the group homes in your area (see Chapter 24).

During your visits, tour the facility and observe the social activities of residents. Talk with the counselors, the residents, and their families. Ask to see a schedule of field trips and daily activities at the home. Discuss how you, your spouse, and your son or daughter feel about each visit. No one home is likely to seem perfect to everyone, especially if you are accustomed to an upper middle class lifestyle. Consider the opportunities for growth that such groups can present for your son or daughter, give extra weight to any preferences he or she might express, and then make an informed and responsible decision as a family.

After a decision has been made, everyone must be committed to making it succeed. As in any separation between a child and a parent, episodes of homesickness and anxiety may occur. Frequent communication can take place by telephone or letter. Be careful not to interfere with the child's adaptation to the new situation by visiting too frequently or taking the child home during periods of loneliness or unhappiness. You can follow your child's progress by calling the home counselors. Try to work out any problems your child reports or you observe by discussing them with the counselors rather than by intervening yourself.

By giving your child the chance to assert her strengths and adaptability, you can ensure the success of a group living situation. The result will be a fuller and more enjoyable life for your adult child and increased peace of mind and pride for you and your spouse. This is worth a slight increase in risk of injury or seizures that comes with less intense, personal supervision.

Maximizing the Independence of an Adult Child Living at Home

If the family decides to have an adult child live with parents, it is important to encourage as much independent living and responsibility as is reasonable for the person to assume. If parents continue to treat an adult child the same way they did when she was an adolescent, the child will probably experience little emotional and psychological growth. Every effort must be made to increase the person's self-esteem and self-reliance.

An adult child living at home can be helped to feel more like an independent adult if she is given freedom to create a home within the home. For example, depending on the parents' resources, a room or section of the house, such as a finished basement or attic, can be turned into an apartment. Parents should regard this area as a separate home. Likewise, the adult child should be responsible for decorating it and keeping it clean. She should also learn to budget money from paychecks or disability payments for room and board, clothes, and entertainment. This type of home situation increases an adult child's confidence and parents' comfort with the idea of moving away from home at some point.

An adult child living at home should be encouraged to find ways to socialize with other adults. Opportunities may be found through epilepsy support groups or community and church activities. A capable child can also volunteer at various organizations. The more she interacts with others as an individual, the more the adult child with epilepsy will be able to develop into a happy, independent adult.

Maintaining a Healthy Parent-Adult Child Relationship

Regardless of the severity of a child's epilepsy, parents can develop healthy and rewarding adult relationships with the child. Open communication about each individual's needs and desires is crucial to allow the relationship to change and mature as the child ages. Good epilepsy care and professional advice can help solve problems or disagreements that may develop regarding the child's independent abilities and the ways that parents provide support. The important goal is for parents and the adult child to live well, with the impact of epilepsy on their relationship minimized as much as possible.

CHAPTER 20

ARE SEIZURES
REALLY THE PROBLEM?

There is an old vaudeville joke about a drunken man looking for his keys under a lamp post (because that is where there was enough light to see by) rather than a hundred feet down the street, where he actually dropped them. The history books tell us that physicians tried to treat George Washington by bleeding and cupping when the real problem was that he was choking to death from tonsillitis. All of this is to introduce questions that every parent of a child with seizures should ask themselves at some time. Are the seizures really my child's big problem? Will things really be different if the seizures are controlled? Is something else going on that I am not dealing with appropriately?

Epilepsy is a disturbance of behavior caused by brain damage. Most commonly, the brain damage is subtle and limited and people with a seizure disorder are as normal as anyone else. However, sometimes the seizures are the result of more severe brain damage affecting a large part of the brain. In those instances, the child with epilepsy not only has seizures, but also has many of the symptoms that can loosely be called mental retardation, cerebral palsy, learning disorders, attention deficit defect, and even, with quite a stretch, autism. These children with multiple handicaps frequently have severe seizure disorders. Often the best that can be achieved by treatment is reduction of the frequency and severity of the seizures, and complete seizure control may not be possible. Even if complete seizure control is achieved, control may have been purchased at the price of severe sedation, ataxia, and difficulty in thinking.

All physicians have encountered parents who, for one reason or another, are unable to accept with any degree of psychological comfort the fact that their child is multiply handicapped. These parents often believe that everything would be fine and the child would be completely normal if only the seizures were completely controlled. I have seen such parents go from physician to physician, experiencing increased frustration with each failure. They often blame the problem on "uncaring" physicians who have actually used the best medical judgment possible in trying to achieve a balance between seizure control and too many side effects.

Each family has its own set of values. For myself, I would rather have a child with occasional seizures who is relatively alert and able to participate in life than a child whose seizures are under control at the cost of being a "zombie." However, that argument can actually be understood only by parents who accept the fact that once permanent brain damage has occurred, the physician may not be able to "fix it."

A similar situation exists with children (and adults) who are not succeeding in life because of a variety of psychological and psychiatric issues. They may be unable to relate well to other people, they may have a short temper, they may be unduly demanding of attention, their style may make other people anxious, and they may not follow through with duties in a responsible manner. In other words, they may suffer from one or many of the problems that interfere with interpersonal relationships for anyone. These psychological and psychiatric problems can be caused by a variety of physical and emotional problems. They must be investigated, diagnosed, and treated as carefully as the seizure disorder itself. Unfortunately, all physicians have encountered patients who tell them that they are discriminated against at work or at school or cannot make friends because they have epilepsy. That may indeed be the situation in some instances. Often, however, the person who is complaining (or the parent who is complaining) is unable or unwilling to accept the fact there are behavioral issues that cause trouble, which would continue to cause trouble whether or not the patient had seizures.

We cannot reverse the problems caused by diffuse brain damage by controlling seizures. We cannot make someone pleasant, attractive, responsible, or comfortable to be around by controlling seizures. We cannot cure George Washington of tonsillitis by bleeding and cupping.

Once again, if the patient is not responding to treatment, then either the diagnosis is wrong, the treatment is wrong, or the patient is not complying with the treatment. Let's be careful to make sure we have a correct diagnosis and know what is causing the problems we are trying to correct, rather than jumping to the conclusion that the seizures are responsible.

CHAPTER 21

SEXUALITY, SEX, AND BIRTH CONTROL

In general, people with epilepsy grow and develop like anyone else. Some antiepileptic medications may reduce sexual feelings for both men or women if the dosage is high, but epilepsy does not prevent people from feeling and expressing normal emotions and sexual desire.

It is important to remember that there is a wide range of "normal" sexual feelings and a wide range of ages when these feelings begin. If you have concerns about your sexuality, find someone knowledgeable to talk to—a parent or other relative, a physician, a teacher, or a counselor.

Everyone must make decisions about sexuality—how, when, why, and with whom to express these feelings and experience intimate behavior. Friends are the usual source of communication about these decisions. This sharing of feelings and information is important and helpful, but it can also be misleading because even friends tend to exaggerate or bend the truth when talking about sex. Parents and other adults are a good source of information and advice. Some adults are not comfortable talking about sex with their own children (or even with others). If you find that an adult is not helpful or seems to be uncomfortable talking to you, ask your physician or school counselor to recommend someone with whom you can talk. Gathering good and honest information is the most important and mature step you can take in developing your own sexuality.

When Should I Expect to Become Interested in Sex?

There is no right or wrong age to become interested in sex. Some people become sexually active at a very early age, while some never have sexual intercourse. The important thing is to be your own person, not to succumb to peer pressure, and to resist being leaned on by an older, more aggressive person. Even though you may feel strong sexual drives, they do not have to be acted upon instantly. Wait until the time is right for you and your partner.

The emotions associated with sexual arousal and love are strong. They are frequently overwhelming, especially in the teenage years. Love does not protect you from the realities of life, especially venereal disease and pregnancy. *Please* read the next section.

Sexually Transmitted Diseases (Venereal Disease)

The three joys of sexual love are pleasure, intimacy, and starting a family. The three downsides are sexually transmitted disease, unexpected pregnancy, and emotional exploitation.

We live in an age in which even once obscure sexually transmitted diseases are becoming common. Sexually active adults travel all over the world and take their germs with them. Not all these diseases can be successfully treated with antibiotics. AIDS is uniformly fatal. Until you are in a monogamous (only one partner) relationship in which both of you are virgins or have tested negative for AIDS, *do not have intercourse without using a condom.* You should not play with a loaded gun, walk across a freeway at night dressed in dark clothing, or make love without protection. This book is not a sex manual. There are good ones on the market. Read one.

Menstruation

Most girls begin to have their menstrual period between the ages of eleven and fourteen years. Having your menstrual period means that your body is producing eggs and that it is possible to get pregnant. It is a time that is accompanied by major hormonal changes, and therefore it is not uncommon for seizures to get worse during the beginning months of menstruation. Some girls who have simple absence seizures may find that their seizures disappear when they begin to menstruate. For reasons that we do not understand, a small number of women find that their seizures are worse either about the time they ovulate (in the middle of the cycle) or at the time of menstrual flow.

Pregnancy

I hope that pregnancy is not an issue for most of the children who will be helped by this book, but many girls get pregnant unexpectedly and at a young age. There are many things to consider before and during pregnancy for someone who has epilepsy. This topic is discussed in greater detail in *Living Well with Epilepsy* (New York: Demos Vermande, 1996).

Every young woman should be aware of the possibility of having a malformed baby as the result of taking medications. Some are more likely to cause trouble than others. Two antiepileptic drugs, valproate (Depakene® or Depakote®) and carbamazepine (Tegretol®), carry a fairly significant risk of spina bifida and other serious malformations that physicians call neural tube defects. Babies born with such a defect may not be able to walk or control their bladder, and some are mentally retarded. Approximately one percent of the babies born to mothers taking valproate have this problem, and about one-tenth to one-half of one percent of the babies born to mothers taking Tegretol® develop it. The risk of this problem becomes much greater if Depakote® and Tegretol® are taken together, and especially if phenobarbital is added to the mix. However, in the last few years, we have discovered that the problem can be reduced substantially, although not completely eliminated, if women who are capable of having children take 800 micrograms (0.8 milligrams) of folic acid (one of the B vitamins) each day. The average over-the-counter multivitamin pill for pregnant women contains 400 micrograms. One of these pills, taken twice a day, provides protection for nearly everyone who is taking ordinary doses of antiepileptic medications. If you are planning to get pregnant, I recommend taking 3 milligrams of folic acid a day for two months before unprotected sex, and to continue to take it throughout pregnancy.

Birth Control

The most effective form of *temporary* birth control (so that you can have a baby if and when you want one) is to regulate the woman's hormones with birth control pills, injections, or implants. No woman should use this form of birth control without first consulting a physician or birth control clinic, having an appropriate examination, and getting an individualized prescription. Birth control pills and these hormones have little, if any, effect on seizure control. Using birth control does not make seizures worse. However, antiepileptic drugs can speed up the metabolism of birth control pills. For that reason, most women taking antiepileptic drugs need a slightly stronger pill than the mini-pill most commonly used. Ask your physician. More information is available in *Living Well with Epilepsy* (New York: Demos Vermande, 1996) or *The Epilepsy Handbook* (New York: Raven, 1995)

For people who are just beginning to engage in sex, condoms are the most readily available, affordable, safe, and effective method—if properly used. Every young man and woman should know how to use the male condom and perhaps even the female condom now that it is available. You are not likely to get good instructions from the boy down the block. Condoms must be used properly to avoid disease and pregnancy. Read the instructions with the package.

Masturbation

Both men and women can masturbate. Most do. Even people who come from a background in which masturbation is considered immoral are likely to masturbate at some time in their life. Long ago there was an old wives' tale that masturbation caused epilepsy or made seizures worse. This is simply not true. In fact, given the pressures and complications of an active sexual life for many people, masturbation may be an appropriate choice to relieve sexual tension. Many people do not have a regular sex partner, have difficulty socially, or simply are not prepared for the emotional and social complications and consequences of having sex with another person. Sexual drive is part of all human beings, and all human beings need the opportunity to gratify this in privacy. Some people who are mentally ill or mentally retarded may not understand when it is appropriate and when it is inappropriate to masturbate. But socializing them about masturbation is no different from socializing them about going to the toilet or eating at the table. It simply takes training.

Impotence

Men with epilepsy must remember that antiepileptic drugs may have effects similar to those of alcohol. Be honest with yourself about your use of alcohol and nonprescription medications. If you think your antiepileptic medications are making it difficult for you to achieve and sustain an erection, talk to your physician about adjusting your medications.

Remember that depression is a common cause of difficulty in enjoying sex. If you are unhappy about yourself, how you are living, and are down on yourself, you cannot be a successful lover. Depression is common and can be treated. Be sure to ask for help.

CHAPTER 22

SLEEP, NUTRITION, AND THE KETOGENIC DIET

All parents want to do what they can to help their children with epilepsy grow and develop well and have fewer seizures. As parents, one of the things we pay most attention to is how our child eats and sleeps. It is important that the child get good nutrition and adequate rest and exercise.

Unfortunately, some parents, in their eagerness to do everything they can, carry things to an extreme. I have seen parents deprive their other children of treats and clothing because they pay exorbitant prices for vitamins and other nutrients at the health food store. In truth, children with epilepsy need proper amounts of ordinary foods and vitamins and these can be obtained at a reasonable cost.

Sleep

Although everyone needs to sleep, people vary in their need for the amount of sleep. If your child is deeply asleep and hard to arouse when it is time to go to school, your child's body is saying it needs more sleep. First you should ask whether the child is getting to bed early enough to feel refreshed. Next, ask your doctor if the sleepiness is caused by toxicity from the antiepileptic drugs. There is no magic number of hours to sleep. Children in general sleep more than adolescents, who sleep more than young adults. Only a few need to sleep more than ten hours a night.

Remember that human beings in general can be divided into morning people, evening people, and mixed. If your child is a night person and doesn't fall asleep until 11:00 P.M., it is not reasonable to expect him to awaken fresh and ready to start the day at 6:00 A.M.! Observe your child and try to figure out his natural rhythm. In general, adult morning people will go to sleep around 9:00–10:00 P.M. and wake up at 5:00 or 6:00 A.M.; night people will go to sleep at 11:00 P.M. to 1:00 A.M. and wake up at 7:00–9:00 A.M. Mixed people will get up early and can function late, but need to rest or sleep sometime in the afternoon. There are of course a very few people at either extreme. Some people get along on four hours of sleep a night and are perfectly content. Some people can't fall asleep before 2:00 or 3:00 in the morning and need to sleep until noon.

Keep a regular schedule, but not necessarily a rigid one. The body doesn't like abrupt severe change. Try to help your child eat three meals a day and go to sleep at a reasonable time each night. That doesn't mean your teenage daughter can't go out to a prom! It means that your teenage son can't get three hours of sleep for three days running.

Nutrition

In general, all your child really needs is a well-balanced diet! In the United States, the newspapers, magazines, and books are filled with diet recommendations. The Department of Agriculture has recently issued a new food pyramid chart, which is a good one to follow. Your local hospital dietitian or the dietitian employed at the local supermarket can help you. Most children with epilepsy are normal children and need normal food. If possible, try to get them accustomed to a relatively lower fat diet with a minimum of sugars and candies. That's just good sense. It has nothing to do with epilepsy, but it will help them become healthier adults. It is important, however, that your child have an adequate supply of fresh fruits and vegetables and enough protein to grow on. This diet need not cost a fortune.

Many people with epilepsy find that caffeine lowers the seizure threshold. Try to limit your child to three cups of weak coffee or three cans of pop a day. It seems to me that the United States is becoming a nation of sleep-deprived people. It is not safe to substitute caffeine for adequate rest.

Even a well-balanced diet may not provide the higher doses of vitamins that we have learned can be helpful. The average child with epilepsy should take one multivitamin tablet a day. This will help insure that they have adequate B vitamins and vitamins A and D. If your daughter is of child-bearing potential, she should take at least 800 micrograms of folic acid a day. This can be obtained by taking two multivitamin tablets that contain 0.4 milligrams of folic acid (400 micrograms), or by taking one prenatal vitamin that contains the same amount of folic acid.

In general, children do not require large additional amounts of vitamins C, E, B6, and so on. There is some evidence that vitamin C (up to 500 milligrams a day in my opinion) and vitamin E (no more than 800 milligrams a day in my opinion) may be helpful in preventing heart disease and stroke in middle-aged people. Some people believe that vitamin C helps prevent colds. Some people believe that higher doses of vitamin B1 (100 milligrams a day) will help keep mosquitoes from biting. None of this relates to epilepsy in particular. Before you have your child take anything more than an ordinary multivitamin each day, be sure to consult with your doctor.

Special Diet

If your child has been diagnosed with phenylketonuria or one of the other inborn errors of metabolism, the diagnosis was probably made because she failed to thrive, developed seizures, or had some other problem. By now, your pediatrician or pediatric neurologist has explained the problem to you and has prescribed a special diet. Take that doctor's advice.

Under no circumstance should a child with epilepsy be given a macrobiotic diet, drink mushroom tea, or use any of the other currently faddish diets and food supplements. Your child with epilepsy is best treated with a generally well balanced diet with modest vitamin supplements.

The Ketogenic Diet

The ketogenic diet suddenly experienced a great surge of publicity in 1994. For hundreds of years, there have been anecdotal reports that people with epilepsy who were starving had fewer seizures. In 1921, Wilder introduced the ketogenic diet as a treatment for epilepsy. The ketogenic diet is actually a controlled form of starvation. It tricks the body into thinking that it is starving, while providing enough calories to permit growth. There are serious problems related to the use of the diet. In an attempt to solve some of the problems, Huttenlacher introduced the MCT (medium chain triglyceride) diet in 1971. This diet is related to the ketogenic diet. It is based on eating large amounts of medium chain triglycerides. It has problems of its own.

The ketogenic diet seems to work best for children between the ages of two and five years. In theory, the diet can be used for all seizure types. Its advocates claim that it works for some patients with complex partial seizures and generalized tonic clonic seizures. However, it has been used primarily to treat medically refractory atonic, myoclonic, and the atypical absence seizures that make up the Lennox-Gastaut syndrome.

If the diet helps the child, it may be very effective and may work for years. If it does not stop seizures within three months, it will probably never be helpful. As many as half of the children on the diet have reported improved seizure control, but only a handful have their seizures completely controlled. The child must remain on the diet for several years, after which is may be slowly tapered until the child can eat a normal diet.

The diet is extremely high in fat, very low in protein, and very low in carbohydrate. It really pushes the extremes. In effect, the patient eats heavy creams and butter.

The diet is very rigid. All food must be weighed and the diet will not work if it is not strictly followed. If the patient does not take specially prescribed vitamins and minerals, he can get very sick. *No sugar is allowed.* Sugar can quickly reverse the beneficial effects of the diet. This means that the diet must be taken under very strict nutritional and medical supervision.

Detailed information about the ketogenic diet can be found in *The Epilepsy Diet Treatment: An Introduction to the Ketogenic Diet,* by John M. Freeman, M.D., Millicent T. Kelly, R.D., L.D., and Jennifer B. Freeman by calling or writing to:

Demos Vermande
386 Park Avenue South, Suite 201
New York NY 10016 U.S.A.
(800) 532-8663
(212) 683-0072

CHAPTER 23

DRIVING
AND EPILEPSY

Earning a driver's license and the freedom to drive an automobile is an important rite of passage for adolescents. For many people, the ability to drive is a crucial part of earning a living, running errands, and pursuing leisure and entertainment activities.

All states restrict the privilege to drive of people with epilepsy, diabetes, heart disease, or other disorders that may cause loss of consciousness. Not being able to drive is often the most frustrating and resented aspect of these chronic diseases. Epilepsy is not nearly as much of a factor in causing automobile accidents as is driving under the influence of alcohol or drugs. But if a person has experienced a seizure in recent months, driving an automobile may be too high a risk, as well as illegal. (Please refer to Appendix 2, "Driving and Epilepsy."

Earning or regaining the privilege to drive can be a major motivating factor for a person with epilepsy to work toward complete control of seizures. If driving is not a reasonable possibility, the person with epilepsy can find pride in learning to use public transportation in order to experience independence to the fullest possible extent. In either case, parents can be a motivating factor and an ally.

Helping Your Child Prepare for Driving Privileges

Everyone should be encouraged to take the classroom part of driver instruction. Even if it seems unlikely at the time that your child will achieve sufficient seizure control to be allowed to drive, it is important to learn the laws of the road and not to be made to feel isolated from other young people.

A good time to begin to assess the possibility of a child with epilepsy being allowed to drive is a year or so before behind-the-wheel driver instruction starts. Let your child know that you are an advocate for driving privileges, not a roadblock.

Bring up the subject of driving at one of your child's regular physician's appointments at the age of 14–15. If your child is having seizures, ask the physician if they will prevent her from receiving permission to drive. Most states require that a person be seizure-free for a certain amount of time and submit a report from their physician on their seizure control and ability to drive safely. The laws about epilepsy and driving vary from state to state, and they change frequently. See Appendix 2 for the most recent summary of state laws compiled by the Epilepsy Foundation of America.

If the physician says that your child's current seizure activity would make driving unsafe, ask for help in improving seizure control. A teenager needs to feel that parents and members of the epilepsy team are there to help her succeed. At the same time, it is important to receive a realistic assessment of the chances of becoming seizure-free and earning driving privileges.

Parents, child, and physician should strive to improve seizure control. If seizures continue despite their efforts, be sure your child is rewarded for trying and is reassured that she is not a failure. If your child has not been evaluated thoroughly at an epilepsy center or is not involved in aggressive antiseizure therapy (involving multiple medications, for example), this is the time to take those steps.

While serving as an advocate for your child, do not attempt to pressure the physician into giving permission to drive. Make sure the physician knows the state laws about driving and epilepsy, and discuss the specific factors contributing to a decision in favor or against granting driving privileges. Some states grant restricted licenses, if recommended by a physician, to allow a person to drive to and from work, within a few miles of home, or in an emergency.

Your child's physician should consider not only whether your child has seizures, but also whether those seizures are likely to cause danger while driving. People who have sudden loss of consciousness without warning are clearly a danger to themselves and others if they drive. But if a person experiences a warning before seizures (an aura) that is long enough to provide time to stop a car, driving might be a possibility. If a person experiences seizures only at night, driving may be allowed during daylight hours in some states. The rules vary greatly from state to state.

Parents and their adult children with epilepsy can help support the Epilepsy Foundation of America (EFA) in its efforts to make the laws that deal with driving and epilepsy more fair. The EFA encourages states to establish medical advisory boards, with at least one neurologist who specializes in epilepsy, to advise them on licensing laws and to mediate requests for driving privileges. This would make it more likely that all people with epilepsy would receive a fair hearing regarding their driving privileges.

Becoming an Advocate for Public Transportation

People who are unable to drive because of epilepsy need to make the most of public transportation and special handi-van services provided to people with handicaps. Parents and the child with epilepsy can become powerful advocates for these services and for expanded public transportation. Don't feel that you are asking for something that you do not deserve because the truth is that automobile drivers use far more public resources and cause more environmental damage than those who rely mostly on public transportation.

Help your child:

- ✧ Continue to drive responsibly while closely following her epilepsy therapy;

- ✧ Work toward better seizure control if she is prohibited from driving; or,

- ✧ Make the most of public transportation and gain pride from living a full life without being able to drive.

CHAPTER 24

INSTRUCTIONS FOR BABYSITTERS

All parents need and deserve some time to themselves, and there will come a time when every child needs to be cared for by someone other than a parent. The technical term for this is "respite care" when someone comes in for an hour, a day, or a year to help care for your child with epilepsy.

Every parent with a child who has seizures should have a copy of the pamphlet "Children and Seizures, Information for Babysitters," published by the Epilepsy Foundation of America (see Chapter 28). The Foundation also publishes a book called *Respite Care*, which contains much useful information.

If you employ babysitters in your home, they need to understand simple first aid, emergency aid, and basic facts about your child's seizure problem. If you have a regular babysitter, he would benefit from reading this book. At the very least, tell your babysitter:

✧ What your child's seizures look like;

✧ The likelihood of your child having a seizure (most children do not have seizures very frequently). Remember that it is quite likely that a child with a seizure disorder will never have a seizure while in a babysitter's care.

✧ What simple first-aid steps the babysitter may need to take. Chapter 11 provides details about first aid for various kinds of seizures.

✧ When and how to call the rescue squad (paramedics). In general, if a seizure lasts more than two minutes, help is needed. The rescue squad also should be called if the seizure happens in water, if the child is not breathing normally after the seizure, if the child vomits during the seizure and does not wake up immediately, or if another seizure starts soon after the first one ends.

✧ How the child acts after the seizure ends and how long it usually takes before he is back to normal;

✧ What medication a child takes; how many times a day it is given; when to give it; how to give it;

✧ Anything the child is not permitted to do;

✧ How to reach you;

✧ Who to call if he cannot reach you;

✧ Anything special about the manner in which the child expresses needs.

If your child has a particularly severe seizure disorder, it may be necessary for you to find one babysitter, preferably an adult, who is interested and willing to learn how to care for the child. It is often easier to find a licensed child care establishment that employs mature adults with whom you can work.

Child care is widely available in some areas and hard to obtain in others. With the passage of the Americans with Disabilities Act, child care programs can no longer discriminate against a child simply because of epilepsy. There are a number of accrediting institutions for child care centers. Two major centers are the National Association for the Education of Young Children, which accredits child care centers, and the National Association for Family Daycare, which accredits in-home or family child care providers.

In order to find an appropriate out-of-home place to care for your child, you need to ask yourself some questions. You should:

✧ Identify your child's needs and the type of care that best meets those needs;

✧ Outline your expectations for your child in the program;

✧ Know how you want your child to interact with other children;

✧ List all activities offered by the program in which you want your child to be included;

✧ Write down any concerns you may have about your child; for example, the need for a special diet or for assistance with feeding;

✧ Specify what, if any, help your child needs with toileting or mobility.

When you visit a child care center to determine if it would be helpful, ask the following questions:

✧ How many children are there per caregiver?

✧ Is the daily schedule structured or nonstructured?

✧ Do the children move from one caregiver to another frequently throughout the day?

✧ Is the environment interesting and stimulating without being overwhelming?

✧ Are there opportunities for your child to have one-on-one time with a caregiver or activities in small groups?

✧ Are you comfortable with the caregiver's philosophy of caregiving?

✧ Is the care centered on children individually or does it focus on peer interaction?

✧ Does the caregiver encourage independence in children?

✧ How are children disciplined?

✧ Does the caregiver interact in a warm, respectful, and appropriate manner?

✧ Is the caregiver willing to communicate with you freely and easily?

✧ Does the caregiver have experience with children who have epilepsy?

✧ What is the daily schedule of activities? What are the nap arrangements?

You should be sure that your caregiver knows the following:

✧ How your child expresses needs;

✧ Your child's motor abilities;

✧ Self-help skills;

✧ How your child interacts with other children;

✧ How your child expresses feelings of frustration, anger, and happiness;

✧ What medication your child takes and the schedule of doses;

✧ Side effects of the medication;

✧ Who is going to give medication to the child;

✧ How to reach you in an emergency;

✧ What constitutes an emergency requiring calling the rescue squad.

All children, including those with epilepsy, have accidents. If you have taken reasonable precautions to find a babysitter or a child care facility, you should not feel guilty if your child has an accident. There is risk in everything we do in life.

CHAPTER 25

RESIDENTIAL FACILITIES

We want to do the very best for our children, particularly if they are sick or handicapped. All too often, however, I see parents who sacrifice themselves, their spouses, and other children in the family in their attempt to help one child who is severely handicapped. Although this is understandable from an emotional point of view, I do not think it is particularly admirable. In fact, the intense focus on the child and the overprotection that usually accompanies it may not be best for that child, to say nothing of its effect on the rest of the family.

It is important that we understand the role of residential facilities for children with epilepsy, especially as parents grow older. Our children usually outlive us, we become weaker as we grow older, and our children have an inborn drive toward independence. Even children who have been overprotected and made overly dependent demonstrate the need for independence by expressions of frustration, temper tantrums, and behavior designed to influence (that is, manipulate) their parents and caregivers. The need for independence becomes a problem as these children reach sexual maturity and enter adolescence. It is always an issue for young adults. Many children and young adults really live more happily in residential facilities than they do at home. Consult with your physician and, equally importantly, with a counselor or social worker if the problems created by caring for a child with severe seizures in your home become something that can no longer be ignored.

This chapter is written from the point of view that you have already decided that residential care is appropriate. Those of you who are wrestling with whether or not to place your child in a residential facility will often need professional help as you come to grips with your individual emotions and circumstances.

When you visit a residential facility, do not expect to find the furnishings and the look of an upper middle class home. Not only is this prohibitively expensive, but it is also usually inappropriate for the needs of young adults with physical handicaps. Rather, be sure that the facility is clean and well lit, with ample space. Look for furnishings along the order of those of a college dormitory.

What to look for:

✦ Are children greeted warmly and helped to feel comfortable?

✦ Do staff members listen and respond to the children rather than simply give directions?

✦ Is there a sensible daily schedule?

✦ What physical activities are there (appropriate to your child's needs)?

✦ What do the children do in bad weather?

✦ Do staff members accept a child's mistakes without getting angry?

✦ Do they limit television viewing time or is it used as a babysitter?

✦ Do they respect and treat each child as an individual (napping, giving medications, diet, toileting)?

✦ Do they look involved and interested rather than bored and tired?

✧ Are reasonable and consistent limits set for behavior?

✧ Do staff members have a sense of humor?

Look around. Are children involved in different activities in the same room?

✧ Do the staff members cooperate among themselves?

✧ Do people seem to be enjoying themselves?

✧ Are activities and play materials suitably adapted for your child's special needs?

✧ Is there an adequate number of staff to meet the needs of the children?

✧ Are there enough toys and furniture?

✧ Are they safe and in good repair?

Ask the following:

✧ When can I visit?

✧ How often are parent meetings and conferences held?

✧ What other types of professional care are available at the facility?

✧ Can physicians and psychologists of my choice, not affiliated with the facility, care for my child?

Review the instructions for babysitters in Chapter 23; the same issues apply in a residential facility.

A word of caution: When residences are good, they can be very, very good. Unfortunately, some of them are just plain awful. The pay scale for workers generally tends to be poor. Supervision by state agencies varies widely. There is no substitute for visiting the facility and seeing for yourself, *but be reasonable*. Be sure to talk with the parents of other residents to find out what problems, if any, they may have encountered. The primary aim of a residential facility is to keep the child clean, comfortable, and safe. Staff members must give medications on time and look for side effects and other illnesses. Independent living skills and other goals of self-fulfillment must be tailored to realistic expectations for each individual child.

Inadequately trained and supervised caregivers can become either unduly anxious or insensitive. Neither is good for the health of your child.

CHAPTER 26

IS IT TIME TO CHANGE PHYSICIANS?

As a child grows and matures, there will be many routine changes in the epilepsy treatment plan. There may also be major decisions to make, such as whether to have surgery, whether to try to withdraw from medications if no seizures have occurred for several years, or whether to seek epilepsy care somewhere else if seizure control is unsatisfactory.

Everyone fears change to some extent, but having the courage and initiative to make a change is often the only way we can improve our lives. This chapter includes suggestions about what to do if things are not going well.

Are You Happy with Your Child's Epilepsy Care?

If your child is having seizures or experiencing undesirable side effects from medications, you should frequently evaluate whether everything possible is being done to stop seizures completely. Your physician and the other members of the epilepsy team should have a clear, well-conceived strategy to reach the goal of *no seizures and no side effects*. It should be a treatment plan that involves you and your child. If it does not, it is time to find a new team.

Here are some questions to ask yourself about your child's care:

❖ Has your child received a thorough diagnostic evaluation? Have you been told what the diagnosis is, what type of seizures are being treated, and what is causing the seizures?

❖ Have you received thorough education about epilepsy in general and how to care for your child in particular?

❖ Do you and your child feel like important parts of the epilepsy care team? Are you asked about preferences or suggestions in planning your child's therapy?

❖ Did your child's physician or nurse explain why a certain medication has been prescribed, why it is important to take it at the prescribed times, and what changes can be made to improve epilepsy control?

❖ Does your child's physician make medication adjustments or follow up with tests or other steps when you report that your child is continuing to have seizures?

❖ Do you go to visits prepared with a detailed seizure log-book and a list of questions or concerns to discuss with the physician and nurses?

❖ Are you and your child following the physician's prescription closely and doing whatever you can do to prevent seizures (such as not allowing the child to become over-tired)?

❖ Have you expressed your dissatisfaction to your physician or nurse? Have they dealt with this forthrightly?

❖ Are you experiencing other problems as a family, or is your child experiencing social problems because of epilepsy?

If, after considering these questions, you are not convinced that everything possible is being done for your child, it is time to make a change. If your child is missing doses of medication or otherwise not following the physician's instructions, ask the nurse how you can improve compliance. Ask the physician if blood tests or other diagnostic tests can be done to provide information that would help improve seizure control. Perhaps more frequent visits and more aggressive therapy would help.

There are three common reasons for a child to continue to have seizures despite treatment with antiepileptic medications: (1) the diagnosis is wrong, (2) the treatment is wrong, or (3) the treatment is right but the child is not receiving it as prescribed. You and your child's physician need to work together to investigate each of these possibilities and to make changes in the child's therapy as they are indicated. Only in a minority of cases do children have seizures that cannot be controlled with existing antiepileptic medications. Even in these cases, new medications are discovered and marketed each year that can be used to try to control the child's seizures.

Ordinary seizures are controlled by ordinary doses of the usual antiepileptic medications. Family physicians should have seizures under control in three months or so. Otherwise, they should refer the patient to a neurologist or directly to a comprehensive epilepsy center if one is nearby. Your physician or nurse should be able to tell you if there is one in your area, or you can call the National Association of Epilepsy Centers (612-525-1160) or the Epilepsy Foundation of America (1-800-EFA-1000) for help. If a neurologist does not have seizures under complete control within six months to one year, make a trip to a comprehensive epilepsy center. It will be worthwhile.

If your child or other family members are experiencing psychological or social problems because of epilepsy, consider seeing a counselor, psychologist, or social worker. Your physician or the local chapter of the Epilepsy Foundation of America (call 1-800-EFA-1000) can recommend counselors who are skilled at helping people with epilepsy and their family members. They can also recommend support groups for children with epilepsy and their parents. These groups can help parents and children overcome the feeling that they are alone in coping with epilepsy, and valuable suggestions and referrals may be obtained from other families.

Intervene Early, As Often As Necessary

The key to helping your child live well with epilepsy is teaching her never to accept anything but the best and to be willing to work hard to get it. Do not tolerate health professionals or others who may try to convince you that things are not that bad or that nothing more can be done. There is almost always something that can be changed, but it takes someone who is willing to make a decision and push for change.

By involving your child in this aggressive pursuit of living well, she will develop the strong self-esteem that will help prevent the problems of social isolation that can affect people with epilepsy.

As we enter a new era of medical care, in which the structure and systems will be completely different from what we have been used to, parents and people with epilepsy must be particularly alert. Quietly sitting back and expecting a physician to do everything possible to assist you is no longer an effective strategy. You must demand aggressive treatment, which may be discouraged because it costs money. Many factors can interfere with your receiving the care that you should.

When You Are Forced to Change Physicians

More and more people find that they must suddenly find a new physician because their employer has contracted for health care from a different health service group (HMO or PPO). This is particularly unsettling when you have a child with epilepsy and need special and often specialized help. If this could happen to you, talk to the person in your company who buys health insurance and express your concerns before they make their decisions for the following year. It is best to talk to them no later than July. Ask your human resources people if provisions can be made for you to have more choices. If not, as soon as you know you must change physicians, start interviewing prospective physicians about their knowledge and interest. If your new plan requires a "gatekeeper"—a family practitioner who must approve your request to see a specialist—interview prospective family physicians carefully. Find one who appreciates your special needs and is willing to help you find an epileptologist.

If you encounter barriers that prevent your child from receiving the care that you believe is necessary, talk first to your physician and then to your employer. Your employer is writing the check and setting the rules. Do not take "no" for an answer.

When Your Child Is No Longer a Child

Pediatricians and pediatric neurologists usually limit their practice to children under the age of sixteen (sometimes eighteen). If your older child has active epilepsy, your pediatric neurologist will ordinarily refer you to an adult neurologist. Ask for several names and ask if there is an epileptologist in your community. Interview prospective physicians about their knowledge and interest in treating young adults with seizure disorders.

CHAPTER 27

CAREER CHOICES FOR PEOPLE WITH EPILEPSY

Children deserve the opportunity to fulfill their ambitions and potential. Every parent has the responsibility to give each child the opportunity to develop ambitions and to provide support to help them reach their goals.

All children with epilepsy can grow up to be active adults with many interests. Most will become employed in vocations and careers, with the potential to be leaders in our society. For those few people whose epilepsy prevents them from holding a regular job, there are other opportunities to stay active and fulfilled.

Considerations About Employment

When considering career or job opportunities, it is important to emphasize what the person *can* do, not the options that may be closed because of epilepsy or other factors. Career planning should begin during junior high school, with help from vocational counselors at school or private agencies. You can encourage your child's interests in science, math, music, and art even in elementary school.

Everyone who desires and *strives* to achieve the highest possible academic and occupational goals should be encouraged. This is especially true for adolescents and young adults, but it also applies to individuals of any age. Today it is common for people to change jobs and even careers several times during their lives. People with epilepsy are no different in this regard. They need to remain aware of changing circumstances — improved seizure control, new training programs, or new technologies that may make it possible to pursue a desired educational or vocational program.

Only a few occupations are ruled out by epilepsy. For example, military service may be a problem. Public transportation careers are also closed to anyone who has experienced loss of consciousness for any reason. This includes being an airplane pilot, train engineer, bus driver, or interstate trucker.

Other occupations may be possible, depending on an individual's seizure control. For example, it may be unsafe for a person who has occasional or frequent seizures to operate dangerous machinery, be a police officer or fire fighter, operate amusement park rides, serve as a lifeguard, be an air traffic controller, or drive a vehicle for a living. Less obvious safety concerns may arise in such situations as being a deep-fry cook at a restaurant or painting houses.

The important thing is to focus on the individual's seizure type and frequency, not simply on the fact that he has epilepsy. Your epilepsy team and an employment counselor can help you and your child evaluate what types of occupations he is interested in and could do safely. Remember that there are many professional occupations that your child can prepare for through higher education. People with epilepsy work as teachers, physicians, nurses, pharmacists, scientists, lawyers, musicians, engineers, or run their own business.

Applying for a Job

If your child is turned down for a job, you can help determine whether epilepsy was the reason and whether fair hiring practices were followed. The following are some ways you can help your teenager or adult child apply for jobs.

Help your child prepare a neat and professional-looking resumé of education, training, previous jobs, explanation of the type of job being sought and why it is of interest, and references from unrelated individuals familiar with the person's personal and job-related characteristics (first ask these people if they would be willing to speak to employers if called). Also ask your child's physician to speak to potential employers on his behalf (you need to give written permission for the physician to release information about your child's health).

Some people think that a resumé is only important when applying for professional positions, but a well-prepared resumé shows any employer that the person is serious about finding a job. A completed job application is still necessary, but the resumé can be sent in advance or attached to the form to give the employer more information about you.

Discuss with your child how best to present the fact that he has epilepsy. If you decide to make it part of the resumé, include an explanation of how seizures are controlled and that they should not interfere with the job requirements. In general, it is best to wait to discuss epilepsy during an interview. Help your child rehearse ways of discussing this in a positive way, such as "I am especially good at assuming responsibility because of the discipline I've learned from taking medications and having a healthy lifestyle in order to prevent my epileptic seizures." By being honest about seizure frequency and type, but also confident about ability to do the job, your child will increase his chances of being hired and succeeding in the job.

The three big determinants of whether or not people get a job are education (are they qualified to do the job?), appearance (do they look neat and clean, like someone the employer would like to represent him?), and attitude (are they eager to help and looking for ways to make a positive contribution?).

We live in an era in which there are many more people than jobs. Employers choose among applicants for a variety of reasons. Don't blame epilepsy if your child is not hired. It is just as likely that she was not qualified in the first place or did not come across as someone who would be a valued employee. Remember that anyone who has the self-discipline, energy, and gumption to deal with epilepsy and to learn to lead a normal life should be an outstanding employee. Try to help your child go into the interview feeling upbeat.

Obtaining Special Training

The Epilepsy Foundation of America has developed a service for helping people with epilepsy to obtain training and find employment. Called the Training and Placement Service, or TAPS, it is funded by the Department of Labor. TAPS representatives work with applicants and their potential employers to help answer any questions the employer or other employees may have about epilepsy and to help the person with epilepsy feel comfortable and work safely in the workplace.

TAPS can provide vocational counseling, help an individual set goals, make career choices, and carry out a job search. It can also put a person with epilepsy in touch with other people who have epilepsy and have found jobs. It can help to have a mentor in a chosen occupation or to discuss the challenges faced in the workplace by people with epilepsy. After a person finds a job, TAPS is available to help with any problems or concerns the employer or employee may have.

The Rehabilitation Services Administration of the United States government provides vocational rehabilitation in every state. Its goal is to help people whose disorder or disability limits the type of work they can do, but who could work if they received vocational training. High school counselors or your local EFA affiliate can refer your child to the state agency that offers this service.

Alternative Forms of Employment

If your child is unable to find a job, consider the possibility of his doing some kind of work out of the home. With computerization and telephone networking expanding the types of work that can be done anywhere, home-based jobs are becoming increasingly common. Other types of work that can be done at home include handicrafts, artwork, writing, telephone marketing, mailing services, and many others. Check your local library for books on home-based businesses.

Another way for a person with epilepsy to gain the self-respect that comes from working is to volunteer at a local charitable organization. This can be an excellent way to socialize with other people, perform valuable services, and even gain experience and references that can lead to a paying job.

There are many employment options for the person with epilepsy who refuses to be limited by the perceptions of others. You can help your child set his sights on obtaining the education and skills that will provide flexibility and enrichment throughout life.

CHAPTER 28

PROTECTING YOUR CHILD'S LEGAL RIGHTS*

The recently passed Americans with Disabilities Act is a good example of how far our society has come in recognizing the rights of people with chronic disorders and disabilities. It is also a recognition of the value each individual has to contribute to society.

As your child grows up, you can make sure that she receives the full educational and career opportunities, government services and assistance, and other rights granted by state and federal laws. These laws change often, sometimes in minor ways that nonetheless may be valuable or create a serious problem for you and your child. If you know your rights and those of your child with epilepsy, you can work against discrimination and stereotypes of people with epilepsy while helping your child fulfill her potential.

This chapter describes some of the legal rights emphasized by the Epilepsy Foundation of America (EFA) in its publications and lobbying of government officials.

*This chapter is based in part on information contained in "The Legal Rights of Persons with Epilepsy," published by the Epilepsy Foundation of America. Contact EFA for updates by its legal department.

Know the Law, Then Use It

Even though we have laws to protect people against discrimination, there is still much discrimination based on race, gender, and disability. To work against that discrimination, each of us needs to understand the laws that apply in each case and then use those laws to protect our rights against those who are either ignorant or defiant of them.

Many laws are difficult to read and understand, and there is often substantial room for interpretation. If you think your child's rights are being denied, first find out about the applicable state and federal laws from your local EFA affiliate and government agencies. Then consider consulting a lawyer. Be sure to find out how much it will cost to discuss your questions for a brief time, such as a half hour. Most lawyers will advise you of your rights and the merits of your case for $50 to $200. If you and the lawyer decide to pursue the matter further, the lawyer will explain how much it is likely to cost. If you have a low income, your state bar association (lawyers' professional association) or law school may be able to refer you to a lawyer who donates time working "pro bono," which in Latin means "for good."

Your Child Is an Individual, Not an "Epileptic"

The most important general right that people with epilepsy have is the right to be treated as individuals and evaluated on the basis of their abilities, not on someone else's ideas about people with epilepsy. This right is the basic premise of the Americans with Disabilities Act: employers and providers of services must make reasonable attempts to accommodate the needs and abilities of each individual. As more people with epilepsy and other disorders are hired and helped to become full participants in our society, biases and stereotypes will be broken down, and we will all be richer because of it.

Insurance and medical care are other areas in which questions of legal rights often arise. In addition to the information provided in

Chapter 24, two legal factors need to be understood. First, a physician is under no obligation to *begin* treating a person (even one who is having a seizure), but once treatment has started it must be continued until the immediate problem is controlled or arrangements have been made for another physician to take over or for you to be given reasonable time, usually two weeks, to find another physician. Second, publicly owned medical centers must treat anyone who requires medical care. The quality of care provided at a county or city medical center is often as good or better than care at private clinics and hospitals.

If you do not feel that your child's medical care has been adequate, first discuss it with the physicians or nurses who provided the care. If you are still dissatisfied (for example, if you don't feel your child has received a complete diagnostic evaluation to identify the cause and type of seizures), request a second opinion. Be aware, however, that unless you have insurance that covers the second opinion, you will probably have to pay for it yourself. Other possible ways to remedy the situation include filing a complaint with the institution's management, with the local medical association, or with a court of law.

In addition to the right to public medical care, people with epilepsy have rights of access to other types of services, such as public transportation, public programs, and any public or private facility open to the public. Most providers of services will happily accommodate special needs if they are contacted in advance. If you believe that your child has been denied access to any type of service or facility because of epilepsy, contact the office of your state attorney general or a lawyer.

What Rights Does a Person Have If Arrested or Searched?

Someone having a seizure may be thought by police or the public to be drunk or under the influence of street drugs. This misperception may lead to the person's being detained, searched, questioned, and arrested. The best way your child can protect against this is to wear a medical identification bracelet or carry medical information in a wallet or purse.

Some states require police to search for medical identification if a person is unconscious or semiconscious. Some states give police and physicians the right to search for medical identification if a person is injured or disabled or behaves strangely in public, and then require that arrangements quickly be made to contact a physician listed on the identification or to transport the person to a safe and appropriate place.

Another legal problem may arise if your child carries an antiepileptic medication in a nonprescription container at school or in public. This medication may be mistaken for illegal drugs, causing school officials or the police to seize them (which could lead to a seizure if the child is denied the medication). This problem can be prevented by fully informing school officials about any medication your child needs to take during the school day. If it is not practical to carry the medication in its prescription container, make sure your child has a copy of the prescription in a wallet or purse. Your pharmacist can give you a small, properly labeled bottle that can be conveniently carried.

How Does Epilepsy Affect Adoption or Child Custody Rights?

Epilepsy may become a consideration in an adoption or child custody proceeding for two reasons:

1. If an adult has epilepsy, it might be a factor that is considered in evaluating parenting ability;

2. It is more difficult to find adoptive homes for children with epilepsy.

In terms of an adult's ability to adopt a child or gain custody, no laws specifically cite epilepsy as a factor in determining fitness to be a parent. The main consideration is to provide for the child's best interests, which includes the adult's ability to provide for the child's emotional and physical needs. Epilepsy may become a factor if the adult's health is greatly affected, but the court must consider the individual's ability to conduct her life and to care for a child.

If you have chosen to adopt a child with epilepsy, you should be aware of state and federal adoption assistance programs that provide financial assistance to parents who adopt such "hard to place" children. Only California still has a state law that allows adoptive parents to petition to annul an adoption if, within five years of the adoption, the child has symptoms of a severe disability that existed without their knowledge before the adoption.

What Educational Rights Does My Child Have?

The Education for All Handicapped Children Act (P.L. 94-142) provides that handicapped children are entitled to a free, appropriate, public education. States must identify and provide specially trained professionals to evaluate children in need of special services. Epilepsy is included as a potential reason for eligibility, but it must be shown that the child's ability or performance in school is adversely affected by the disorder. Individual instruction provided early and by a teacher trained to help overcome learning disabilities related to epilepsy can help a child achieve maximum educational potential.

An important part of this federal law requires that, whenever possible, handicapped children be educated with children who are not handicapped. This is often referred to as "mainstreaming" and can help a child with epilepsy adjust to the disorder and develop good self-esteem. It also helps teachers and other children understand and accept disabilities and disorders such as epilepsy. However, a mainstreamed child may not be able to get the individual attention she needs to learn.

Every child is entitled to a free public education through high school. Higher education is not free, but federal law requires that admission procedures be fair and that people with disabilities have access to all facilities and educational opportunities at a college or university. Few state colleges and universities even ask if a prospective student has epilepsy. Those who ask about epilepsy or other medical conditions report that this information is used to identify medical needs of students. The EFA believes that such information should be provided voluntarily, if at all, and must be kept confidential and not used as a basis to deny admission. Students with epilepsy may want to provide relevant information to the student health service in case they need assistance while at school. Also, some colleges have a student epilepsy support group that may help your child overcome any problems she might encounter on campus.

Can an Employer Refuse to Hire Me Just Because I Have Epilepsy?

If your child is not hired, review the application process and interviews, if any were held, and make a list of qualifications, hiring criteria, special job requirements, and questions asked and statements made by the interviewer. Then decide together whether the process was fair. Remember that legitimate safety issues, requirements for the job, and applicants who were more qualified are legitimate reasons why your daughter might not have been hired.

If you and your child decide that the process was not fair, do *not* immediately write or call the employer with accusations of unfairness or discrimination. Instead, help your child (if necessary) write to the employer, asking politely for information about the hiring decision so that she can learn how to improve chances for future opportunities with that employer. Doing this in writing and keeping copies of all correspondence are important ways to document any complaint you might decide to make.

If the employer refuses to answer the inquiry or if the answer does not seem honest compared to statements made in the interview, follow up with a letter mentioning the Americans with Disabilities Act and citing questions or concerns you have with the hiring practice. Ask for another interview to allow your child to present further evidence that epilepsy does not interfere with her ability to do the job. Ask the employer to call your physician to discuss whether epilepsy will interfere with your child's ability to do the job safely and well.

If the employer still refuses to consider your requests for more information or responds in ways that you and your child think are inadequate, consider filing a complaint with your county or state equal employment opportunity office. More information about employment rights and legal advice can be obtained from the Epilepsy Foundation of America (EFA). See Chapter 29 for how to contact the EFA and other resources.

The Americans with Disabilities Act requires that employers make a reasonable accommodation for an employee who is disabled. It does not relate at all to dependents of the employee. The employer cannot inquire about disability until after a conditional offer of employment is made and a medical examination is requested. At that point, you are obliged to discuss it with a physician who is doing the examination. If the employer makes an outright offer of employment and does not require an examination, you are under no obligation to disclose your disability; you were not asked.

The Equal Employment Opportunity Office is a state office that operates under federal law to investigate alleged discrimination for age, protected status (such as race, sex, or religion), or disability.

The Family Emergency Medical Leave Act

This is potentially the most important piece of modern legislation for the parent of a child with seizures. It has no relationship whatsoever to the Americans with Disabilities Act, and relates primarily to caregivers of someone in the family who is sick. The regulations are rather complicated and all I can do is outline a few of the main points.

The FEMLA relates to employees of employers who have fifty or more employees within a seventy-five mile radius. The employee must have worked for twenty or more consecutive work weeks, not counting sick leave or vacation, and must have been employed for at least twelve months. Before the leave begins, the employee must have worked 1,250 hours prior to the start of the leave. Sick leave and vacation do not count; these are actual hours worked. An employee is allowed to take twelve work weeks of unpaid leave (the employer may pay for it under certain circumstances if they chose). The twelve weeks may or may not include sick leaves or other uncompensated leave, depending upon the policies of each individual employer.

An employee can request leave under the FEMLA in order to:

1. Care for a newborn child, a child placed with the family for adoption, or a child placed with the family for foster care within twelve months of the date the child becomes your responsibility. Either the husband or the wife can request the leave.

2. The employee may take the leave to care for a spouse, parent, or child with a serious health condition. Parent is defined as anyone who raised you when you were a child, not just blood parents.

A serious health condition is an illness, injury, or impairment, either physical or mental, which involves either inpatient care or is the result of outpatient care of more than three continuous days of treatment, requiring continuing treatment by a health care provider. Continuing treatment means two or more visits beyond the initial three days.

The time off can be taken full-time, on a reduced schedule, or intermittently, e.g., every six weeks to help someone go through chemotherapy.

The employer may require back to work certification. The employer may require thirty days notice if you know before a child is due to be delivered or if the treatment is being planned in advance. Under FEMLA, the employer can ask about disability. You are obliged to disclose the disability to the extent it is job-related or the information is consistent with business necessity. The employer may not ask questions about any future conditions.

A number of states also have parenting leave laws, which vary broadly.

The Family Emergency Medical Leave Act and the Americans with Disabilities Act are relatively new laws, which are undergoing rapid change. If you encounter any problem in getting the help you need from your employer, you probably should consult an attorney who is experienced in labor law.

Can Epilepsy Cause Criminal Behavior?

Studies show that the prevalence of epilepsy among people in prisons and jails is approximately three times greater than in the general population. This does not, however, mean that epilepsy causes violence or other criminal behavior, as was once thought. Rather, three sociological factors have been identified:

1. Due to the stigma associated with epilepsy and society's frequent rejection of persons who have the condition, some people with epilepsy have difficulty adjusting socially, which may result in hostile or antisocial behavior.

2. People who are involved in criminal activity are more likely to have been physically abused or to be alcohol abusers, both of which can cause a person to develop epilepsy.

3. People with epilepsy may experience learning, thinking, and/or employment difficulties and may therefore be among those of lower socioeconomic status who are more likely to be imprisoned for their acts.

Can a Person with Epilepsy Be Committed Involuntarily to a Mental Health Facility?

No state allows commitment based solely on a person's epilepsy, and the involuntary commitment laws of most states are limited to people who are mentally ill or mentally retarded. Even in these cases, the state must usually show that the person is a danger to himself or to others or is incapable of self-care. The EFA does not believe that epilepsy is a reason to take an individual's freedom away, and that even when epilepsy is accompanied by mental illness or mental retardation, involuntary commitment should be the last resort. If commitment is necessary, every effort should be made to protect the rights of the person and to guarantee continuing medical treatment according to accepted standards.

Several states allow the parents or guardians of a person with epilepsy to temporarily admit that person to a respite facility, even if the person with epilepsy does not want to stay there. The intent of this is to allow the parents or guardians time to rest from the requirements of providing care for the person. The time limit for this respite care ranges from twenty-one to thirty days.

Can People with Epilepsy Be Denied Housing or Loans?

The Americans with Disabilities Act prohibits discrimination in housing based on handicaps and disorders such as epilepsy. It also prohibits the denial of access to public transportation to handicapped persons. Because the ADA is a relatively new law, many renters and lenders are not aware of their obligations to consider people with epilepsy equally and without discrimination. Also, parts of the law are vague and you may need legal interpretation or assistance in protecting the rights of your child and family. Contact a lawyer or the state human rights commission if you feel your child has been discriminated against in any of these areas.

How Can I Help Protect and Extend the Rights of People with Epilepsy?

Despite improvements in state and federal laws, discrimination against people with epilepsy is still a major problem. In fact, these discriminatory acts sometimes cause more problems than the disorder itself. You can help improve the quality of life for everyone with epilepsy by knowing the laws in your state, county, and city, and by being willing to take whatever steps are necessary to protect your rights and those of your child. Support the efforts of and contribute financially or through volunteer work to national, state, and local offices of the EFA. Your family can help continue the progress that has been made in recent years.

A worthwhile book is *A Guide to Legal Rights for People with Disabilities*, Marc D. Stolman (New York: Demos, 1994).

CHAPTER 29

OBTAINING HEALTH INSURANCE

Although the United States offers the best health care in the world, not everyone has access to it. This is a national disgrace. Efforts to develop and fund a national health care plan have failed in the U.S. Congress. At present there is no possibility for universal access, meaning that everyone will be guaranteed a fairly broad range of preventive, diagnostic, and therapeutic medical services.

It is not yet clear exactly how a new health care insurance system will be structured, funded, and administered. Its shape will be determined by the individual actions of employers, insurers, and the states. What is not likely to change is the need for families to learn how to use whatever system exists to obtain the best health care possible. It is important to understand how the current system works and be prepared to take advantage and avoid the pitfalls of the new system. One thing has become clear. Managed care plans run by large corporations will become more common, perhaps even the norm.

Everyone will face barriers toward getting comprehensive care. All the plans for new health care systems emphasize the rationing of care and barriers toward the free choice of physician. Having health insurance that will pay the physician is of little use is you can't use it to see the *right* physician. We should all talk to our legislators about being sure that we have free choice of physicians. We will all have to learn to fight our way through the system to get the care we need.

Can People with Epilepsy Get Insurance?

There are many different types of insurance, including health, life, disability, automobile, and home insurance. People with epilepsy can get most types of insurance, but usually not as easily nor as inexpensively as people who do not have medical disorders or diseases, and benefits may be limited. This may not seem fair, but you have to consider that insurance companies must make a profit. They try to make sure that the premiums paid by policyholders for insurance more than cover all future costs the company will incur, including the administrative costs of running the company. Insurance companies face price competition, so their profits are based on reducing costs. The most effective way to do this is to reduce risk, which means turning away the very people who most need insurance.

Insurance companies try to earn a profit by offering insurance at different rates to different groups of people. Their rates are based on the likelihood that a person or family will require payment for covered services, such as medical care, a disability or death benefit, or car repairs. An individual's rates for each type of insurance may depend on factors such as age, current and past health, and driving record. People with epilepsy (and other chronic disorders) are often charged more for health and life insurance than the general population, regardless of how their health is actually affected by the disorder.

This may change if the law prohibits discrimination because of preexisting conditions and a single premium rate for everyone. Insurance companies rarely acknowledge that the long-term health of people with epilepsy and other chronic disorders can be improved by paying for good preventive care and education about self-care, thus saving the insurance company money. It is hoped that some day this preventive, cost-saving approach might become more common throughout the United States, depending on how the law is structured. For this to work, the patient has to stay with the insurance company a long time. But employers buy insurance on price and change companies frequently.

Regardless of what type of insurance you are buying, you have to search for the best insurance for the most reasonable cost. When you obtain price quotes from several companies, be sure that each agent is quoting a rate based on the same type and amount of coverage. This can be confusing, so keep asking questions until you understand. It is the insurance company's responsibility to explain exactly what types of coverage you can buy for how much money. Write down this information and obtain a copy from the insurance agent to compare with types of coverage and rates from others. If you decide to purchase a policy, the insurance company must provide you with a written explanation of exactly what you have purchased. An independent insurance broker can help you with this.

It helps to get to know an individual insurance agent whom you can call with any questions or problems. Make sure you understand when and how you are supposed to send payments (premiums) for the insurance. As the holder of an insurance policy, it is your responsibility to know what your policy covers. You must know how to obtain payment for covered services, and you must file claims according to the procedures set by the company. Sometimes there may be time limits for filing claims, so it is important to obtain and fill out the proper forms promptly. It is also the policyholder's responsibility to pay premiums on a timely basis. Some states require a grace period of ten to fourteen days for late payments. This means that as long as you send your payment within that time, your policy is still in effect. Know the time requirements for your premiums because if you let your policy lapse, you might lose all past and future rights under the insurance.

Before you can shop for insurance, however, you need to know which types are available. The following section describes current types of health care insurance. The type of insurance may differ depending on where you live, and it will almost certainly change over the next few years. As you shop for insurance for yourself and your child with epilepsy, make sure that you think about future needs as well as current ones.

Indemnity or Fee-for-Service Health Insurance

This is the traditional kind of health insurance and gives the policyholder the most freedom of choice. If you have this type of insurance, you can choose to see any private physician at any time, and you can be treated in any hospital you choose. The insurance pays a set percentage (usually 80% of the amount above an annual deductible) of the costs of covered care, and you pay the rest, called a copayment. Claims must usually be filled out and submitted by the policyholder. If you choose this type of health insurance, be sure that care and medications for epilepsy are covered and that you can afford to pay the premium. Often the 20% copayment is limited to a certain amount each year so that there is a limit to how much you have to pay any given year.

Because of the rising costs of health care, indemnity insurance is rapidly being replaced by managed programs of health care, described below.

Health Maintenance Organizations (HMOs)

Health maintenance organizations are a type of health service organization that has grown rapidly since the early 1980s. They actually guarantee to provide a range of services described in a contract. Care is provided by health professionals at participating clinics and hospitals. There are three main differences between indemnity insurance and HMOs.

✧ In an HMO you pay a fixed monthly premium that covers all (or nearly all) of your health care costs without having to submit claims.

✧ An HMO restricts you to seeing certain physicians at certain clinics and hospitals.

✧ The management of the HMO decides what care you will or will not receive.

The theory underlying HMOs is that they can keep costs down by organizing hospitals and physicians and by paying them set amounts according to how many patients they see and the services they provide. Experts expected HMOs to keep costs as low as possible by encouraging policyholders to use preventive services and by competing with indemnity insurance companies and with each other. It is hard to tell if this has happened because the costs of new medical technology and an aging population have caused overall health care costs to rise rapidly despite this competition. In fact, HMOs have tended to price their services just below the competition rather than just above their costs. In most cases HMOs control their costs by avoiding taking on people with preexisting conditions and by limiting the services they provide.

Each type of HMO is organized and operates somewhat differently. These differences can have a drastic impact on people's ability to obtain high quality health care, especially those with chronic disorders. HMOs vary widely in how they restrict members' choices of primary physicians, specialists, clinics, and hospitals.

The most restrictive type is called a "staff-model HMO." It will pay only for services provided by physicians at a clinic owned by the HMO and at a hospital that has a contract with the HMO. In this type of plan, the physicians are employees of the HMO and are usually paid an annual salary plus bonuses according to how many patients they see or how much money the HMO earns that year.

The least restrictive type of HMO is called an "IPA-model HMO." IPA stands for "independent practitioner affiliated," which means that the HMO company signs contracts with private physicians who agree to provide care to its members for set fees, plus some type of annual bonus system. There is a wide range of HMO plans with degrees of member freedom somewhere between the strict staff and the IPA models.

Preferred Provider Organizations

A preferred provider organization (PPO) is a cross between an indemnity plan and an HMO. A PPO plan pays all or most of the costs of services provided by selected physicians and hospitals. The difference is that a PPO allows members to go to other physicians and hospitals if they are willing to pay a portion of the costs, usually 20 percent plus a deductible amount.

A note of caution: HMOs and PPOs are new in some parts of the country and are undergoing many changes. Some have been closed for fraud. Many have gone bankrupt or been merged with other HMOs. This may leave members without coverage or receiving lower quality coverage. Indemnity insurance companies have been providing health insurance for much longer, and few have gone into bankruptcy. Consider these facts when you are choosing among health insurance options offered by an employer or are shopping for insurance on your own.

Medicare

Medicare is a form of health insurance for those over age sixty-five and for younger people who are totally disabled. It is provided and administered by the federal government. There are two parts to Medicare, Part A and Part B. Part A covers services provided in hospitals as well as some nursing home and home-care services for a short time after a patient leaves the hospital. It is financed by employee and employer Social Security taxes. Part B is voluntary health insurance that partly covers physicians fees, clinic visits, diagnostic tests, and some home health visits. It is financed by a combination of monthly premiums paid by those enrolled and a matching amount from government funds.

The coverage provided by Medicare and the costs to those enrolled change every few years, as the government attempts to stretch available funds to meet rising health care costs. Medicare has been severely strained because the average life expectancy is now above seventy-five and many more people are living into their eight-

above seventy-five and many more people are living into their eighties and nineties.

Medicare cannot be relied on for all health care needs; for example, it pays very little for long-term care provided in the home or in a nursing home and medicines are not covered. Access to physicians for patients on Medicare is becoming a problem because it pays the physician only about 50 percent of his or her usual charges.

Medicaid

Medicaid is health insurance for the poor and the near poor. It is funded by a federal subsidy to states, each of which then decides how much state money to contribute and what type of coverage to offer. For this reason, coverage varies greatly in different states, and it can change from year to year based on the financial condition of the state. It pays physicians and hospitals very poorly. Access to good care by Medicaid recipients has become a major problem.

State Health Insurance Risk Pools

Some states have recognized that people with chronic health disorders may be unable to obtain health insurance or must pay very high rates for coverage. To make insurance available to them, some states have passed laws requiring health insurance companies operating in the state to contribute to an organization that provides insurance to those who cannot qualify or who must pay a high price for standard health insurance.

For example, in 1976 Minnesota established the Minnesota Comprehensive Health Association (MCHA), which spreads the costs of high-risk insurance among all health insurance agencies in the state. Anyone is eligible for coverage who has been refused health insurance, whose premiums exceed those available through MCHA, or who has one of the medical conditions covered automatically by MCHA. The plan covers 80% of costs over an annual $1,000 deductible per person, and 100% of costs over a $3,000 deductible per family. A supplement to Medicare is offered for those over age sixty-five. Minnesota has also recently launched two new health insurance initiatives. One provides basic services to children and pregnant women in low-income families. The other, called Minnesota Care, is a drastic overhaul of health care in the state to control costs and provide universal access to basic health care. Studies of the effectiveness and costs of these programs and those in other states will be useful in planning for the future.

If you have been refused health insurance or feel that your premiums are too high, check with your state insurance officer, your insurance agent, or your local office of the Epilepsy Foundation of America to find out if your state offers a pooled risk insurance plan.

WHERE TO TURN WHEN YOU NEED HELP

The organizations listed in this chapter are especially good at helping individuals and their families live well with epilepsy. Contact them for general information, advice, support, health care, and to find out what services are available in your area.

Advocacy and Assistance for People with Epilepsy

The Epilepsy Foundation of America (EFA) (4351 Garden City Drive, Landover, MD 20785; 301-459-3700; toll-free, 1-800-EFA-1000) is the only national, charitable, nonprofit voluntary agency in the United States specifically dedicated to the welfare of people with epilepsy. Approximately one hundred local organizations around the country are affiliated with the EFA. If you do not know the phone number or address of your nearest affiliate, call the toll-free national number.

The EFA national office publishes information and presents educational programs on epilepsy, works with lawmakers to encourage the passage of laws that treat people with epilepsy fairly, and supports epilepsy research. EFA also publishes a monthly newsletter called "Epilepsy U.S.A."

State and local EFA affiliates are usually United Way agencies and offer a range of services and programs depending on the support they receive. Programs may include:

✧ Information and referral services;

✧ School Alert programs to improve the school environment for children with epilepsy;

✧ Self-help groups and parent groups;

✧ Recreational and education programs for young people with epilepsy;

✧ Community education, especially during November, which is National Epilepsy Month;

✧ Educational programs for health care professionals;

✧ Community residences for people with epilepsy who need some help in order to live independently;

✧ Counseling for people with epilepsy and their families;

✧ Advocacy for those who are being discriminated against because of epilepsy;

✧ Job search and employer educational programs (Training and Placement Service).

Health Care for People with Epilepsy

Comprehensive Epilepsy Programs (CEPs)

The development of programs specifically designed for and dedicated to treating and studying epilepsy—CEPs—was spurred by a policy statement from the National Institute for Neurological Disorders and Stroke (NINDS), a part of the National Institutes of Health (NIH). This statement noted in part that "epilepsy is a complicated, chronic disorder and should be treated in a comprehensive way."

Money from the NIH research budget was provided in 1975 to start CEPs in Minnesota (MINCEP® Epilepsy Care), Virginia (University of Virginia Comprehensive Epilepsy Program), and Oregon (Comprehensive Epilepsy Center of Oregon). In 1976, NIH funds were provided for CEPs in Augusta (Georgia Comprehensive Epilepsy Program) and Seattle (Regional Epilepsy Program). In 1980, a CEP opened in Los Angeles (UCLA Urban Comprehensive Epilepsy Program). CEPs were created to provide the best care for people with epilepsy; to serve as a laboratory for multidisciplinary research; to educate doctors, nurses, and other caregivers; and to organize community services.

Only the CEPs in Minnesota and Los Angeles continue to receive NIH funding, and that only for research. This lack of support has reduced services or closed some others. Yet they have proven and some continue to demonstrate the validity of a comprehensive, multidisciplinary team approach to providing epilepsy care. Newer programs to treat epilepsy with modern techniques are developing across the country. They are helping to improve seizure control in many patients with difficult seizures; they are improving the lives of individuals with epilepsy and their families; and they are greatly expanding knowledge of the clinical treatment of epilepsy.

If your child continues to have seizures or is experiencing side effects that make it difficult to think or function in daily life, discuss the problem with your child's doctor or obtain a neurologist's opinion. If your child's seizure control or alertness does not improve, seek help at a CEP. Contact the EFA or the local affiliate for a referral to a reputable program near you. You can also call the National Association of Epilepsy Centers (612-525-4526), which is trying to improve access to and the quality of care offered by epilepsy treatment programs.

Publications and Audiovisual Materials on Epilepsy

The following centers are active in producing educational materials on epilepsy. Some publications are free, but others must be purchased; audiovisual materials usually can be either rented or purchased. Contact them for a current catalog of their offerings.

Epilepsy Foundation of America
4351 Garden City Drive
Landover, MD 20785
301-459-3700; toll-free, 1-800-EFA-1000

MINCEP® Epilepsy Care
5775 Wayzata Boulevard
Minneapolis, MN 55416
612-525-2400

Comprehensive Epilepsy Program
Bowman Gray School of Medicine
Winston-Salem, NC 27103
1-800-642-0500 (toll-free in North Carolina)

Legal Assistance and Information for People with Disabilities

Administration on Developmental Disabilities (ADD)

Write to Room 340E, Hubert H. Humphrey Building, 200 Independence Avenue, S.W., Washington, D.C. 20201 for the location of the nearest ADD office, which can provide specialized help and information on laws and services for people with disabling medical conditions.

Epilepsy Foundation of America

The EFA publishes a comprehensive, up-to-date, loose-leaf binder containing information on federal and state laws pertaining to epilepsy. A pamphlet on the legal rights of people with epilepsy is also available. (See address and phone number earlier in chapter.)

Camps for Children and Teens with Epilepsy

A child whose seizures are well-controlled can probably safely attend any well-supervised, reputable camp for children. Children whose seizures are not necessarily well-controlled or who want to learn more about epilepsy and share experiences with other children with the disorder may benefit greatly from a camp specifically for children with epilepsy. These camps also may offer special programs for teens with epilepsy, as well as an opportunity for the teen to be a counselor for children with epilepsy.

Parents should call the EFA for a list of camps for children with epilepsy. They should then contact the camp director for complete information on the camp's medical staff, educational program, recreational activities, facilities, safety procedures, length and dates of programs, cost, and the age range and medical condition of youth accepted. You and your child may also want to attend an orientation meeting or open house at the camp before deciding whether to attend. Camp Oz in Minnesota (612-646-8763) serves children from all over the United States.

Help for Parents of Children with Chronic Disorders or Disabilities

The National Network of Parent Centers, Inc.

This is a national network of organizations called Technical Assistance for Parent Programs (TAPP). It is funded by the U.S. Department of Education, Office of Special Education and

Rehabilitative Services. TAPP programs provide training and information to parents of handicapped children. They have created an environment in which experienced, knowledgeable parents can help other parents. To find the TAPP in your area, contact the national office or the office for your region.

National Office: Federation for Children with Special Needs, 95 Berkeley Street, Suite 104, Boston, MA 02116; 617-482-2915; 800-331-0688; Fax: 617-695-2939.

Northeast Regional Center: New Hampshire Parent Information Center, P.O. Box 1422, Concord, NH 03302-1422; 603-224-7005; 800-232-0986 (NH only); Fax 603-224-4365 (serves New Hampshire, Maine, Vermont, Connecticut, New York, Rhode Island, Massachusetts, Pennsylvania, New Jersey, Delaware, Maryland, Puerto Rico, and Washington, D.C.).

West Regional Center: Washington State PAVE, 6316 South 12th Street, Tacoma, WA 98465; 206-565-2266; 800-572-7368; Fax 206-566-8052 (serves Washington, Montana, Wyoming, Idaho, Oregon, Alaska, Hawaii, Utah, California, Texas, New Mexico, Arizona, Nevada, Department of Defense Dependents' Schools (DODDS), and The American Territories).

Midwest Regional Center: PACER Center, Inc., 4826 Chicago Avenue, Minneapolis, MN 55417-1098; 612-827-2966; 800-537-2237; Fax 612-827-3065 (serves Wisconsin, Michigan, Ohio, Indiana, Iowa, Illinois, Kentucky, Missouri, Kansas, Nebraska, Minnesota, North Dakota, South Dakota, and Colorado).

South Regional Center: PEP, Georgia ARC, 2860 East Point Street, Suite 200, East Point, GA 30344; 404-761-3150; 800-966-3150; Fax 404-767-2258 (serves Georgia, Arkansas, Louisiana, Mississippi, Alabama, Florida, South Carolina, Tennessee, Virginia, West Virginia, and Oklahoma).

The following organizations for parents and professionals improve the ability of families to provide care for children with special health care needs. They can provide audiovisual materials, publications, technical assistance, and referral to programs in your area.

Association for the Care of Children's Health (ACCH)
7910 Woodmont Avenue, Suite 300
Bethesda, MD 20814
301-654-6549; 800-808-2224; Fax 301-986-4553
An association of professionals and parents that provides written and audiovisual materials as well as consultation services to help people take a family-centered approach to caring for children with special health needs.

Federation for Children with Special Needs
95 Berkeley Street, Suite 104
Boston, MA 02116
617-482-2915; 800-331-0688; Fax 617-695-2939
Administers the Collaboration Among Parents and (Health) Professionals (CAPP) project. This project encourages the involvement of parents in the health care of their children with chronic illness or disability. It also promotes partnerships between parents and health care professionals.

National Maternal and Child Health Resource Center
College of Law Building
The University of Iowa
Iowa City, IA 52242
319-335-9067; Fax 319-335-9098
Provides information, assistance, and training materials to promote the improvement and expansion of maternal and child health services, including services for children with special health care needs.

Community Resources and Social Services

Most cities, counties, and states support an array of social services that provide for financial, educational, vocational, legal, residential, counseling, and transportation needs. It may seem confusing to try to find the services in your area and to gain access to them, but be persistent. If you are not sure where to go for help or do not get the help you need, ask for help from a social worker or from your local EFA affiliate.

If you do not know where to get help, start with your county welfare department or a family social service agency (e.g., Catholic Charities, Jewish Family Service, Lutheran Social Services). They serve people of all races and religions, even those who are not poor. Your local hospital social worker should have a list of resources for your use.

CHAPTER 31

KEEPING HOPE ALIVE THROUGH RESEARCH

The 1990s have been designated by Congress as the "Decade of the Brain." This commitment to brain research recognizes the potential for major advances in our understanding of the brain and our ability to effectively treat brain disorders. This has been made possible by advances made over the past three decades in techniques and tools used to study the brain. By combining new knowledge of genetics, cell biology, structure, function, and behavior, scientists are gaining a better understanding of how the human brain works. This understanding provides the foundation for developing improved methods to prevent, treat, or cure diseases and disorders affecting the brain.

By following the progress of brain research and epilepsy research, you can share in the excitement of new discoveries and the hope for better therapies. However, be cautious when scientific "breakthroughs" are announced in newspapers or on television. These accounts are often exaggerated or sensationalized to attract attention, or they do not provide enough information to help people understand the real significance of the scientific advance. Ask your child's epilepsy team or the EFA if you have questions about an epilepsy research report.

Another way to gain hope from epilepsy research is to improve your understanding of the brain and how research is conducted. This chapter explains different types of research and some of the recent developments related to epilepsy.

For more information about the brain and current research, see the September 1992 issue of *Scientific American*, an excellent special issue on "Mind and Brain." An overview of brain research activities sponsored by the federal government, titled "Maximizing Human Potential: Decade of the Brain 1990–2000," is available from the National Foundation for Brain Research, Suite 300, 1250 24th Street N.W., Washington, DC 20037.

What Are the Different Types of Research?

Research activities can be broken down into three general types: basic science, developmental research, and clinical studies. Each type is important, and all three types are necessary to advance medical care.

Basic Science

Basic science is the search for new knowledge about how things work. Scientists who study the nervous system (neuroscientists) are trying to figure out how the 100 billion neurons (nerve cells) that make up the central nervous system function independently and in networks. They also study brain structure and function to gain a better understanding of how specific parts of the brain control various activities.

Because of the complexity of the human body and other natural systems, basic scientists must focus their investigations on very specific questions. For example, no one scientist would be able to study a question as general as "how does the human brain work?" Neuroscientists must specialize in studying specific parts or features of the nervous system, such as how neurons combine chemistry and electricity to communicate with each other. Even this type of question must be broken down into small parts to be worked on by different scientists because there are several different types of neurons and a wide variety of neuron structures, and each exchanges information differently.

In order to understand how a seizure begins in one part of the brain and spreads to involve millions or billions of neurons, we must understand how each type of neuron communicates with other neurons in the many types of neuron networks within the brain. This is the role of basic science: to provide the fundamental understanding on which to base ideas for preventing or treating diseases and disorders.

As each neuroscientist answers a specific question about the nervous system, he writes an article to be submitted to a research journal. Reputable journals send submitted articles to other scientists in the author's field of research, who review whether the author followed an accepted scientific method of research and analyzed and explained the results of the research accurately. Neuroscientists share their discoveries and build on each other's work through research results published in journals and presented at scientific meetings.

Money to support basic research in the United States comes mostly from the National Institutes of Health (NIH), in Bethesda, Maryland. NIH research is funded by taxpayers' money in amounts decided each year by the President and Congress. Funds for neuroscience research come mostly from a branch of the NIH called the National Institute of Neurological Disorders and Stroke. Funds for basic research are used to buy laboratory equipment and research animals and to pay the salaries of the teams of scientists who conduct the thousands of experiments needed to answer each scientific question. Most of these teams work in universities and are made up of college students, laboratory technicians, recent Ph.D. recipients who are gaining experience in a specialized field, and faculty members who teach and do research.

The purpose of basic science is to explain the physical world and to discover how living things function. A researcher doing basic science research tries to explain things as they are, rather than look-ing for ways to fix things that have gone wrong. However, most of the important scientific breakthroughs have resulted from the dis-covery of how a very small part of a living system functions or is organized. Almost all neuroscience research has potential applica-tions for epilepsy because it provides better understanding of how neurons function and how various brain structures communicate with each other.

We have a very long way to go before we understand how the brain stores memories or directs body functions, but basic science is steadily providing new knowledge about little pieces of this large puzzle. This new knowledge then provides clues for work in the next area of research—developmental research.

Developmental Research

Developmental research is designed to develop the new equip-ment and animal models needed to study diseases and disorders and the new drugs and other therapies needed to prevent, treat, or cure medical problems. Basic science discoveries provide a starting point. For example, physics experiments with different forms of energy led to the development of various types of imaging instruments. New types of microscopes and medical imaging devices have greatly improved the ability of scientists to study the nervous system in the laboratory and clinic.

Although it took about three hundred years to perfect the light microscope with which most people are familiar, it took only twen-ty years to develop an electron microscope capable of photograph-ing structures many thousands of times smaller than can be seen with light microscopes. Electrons have shorter wavelengths than light and can be used to image features of materials or cells magni-fied as little as ten times to as many as five million times. Electron microscopes greatly increased the scientist's knowledge about what is inside cells such as neurons. But a major drawback to using the various types of electron microscope is that the sample to be viewed must be sliced very thin and treated with chemicals. This allows sci-entists to study the structure of cells, but it does not allow them to tell how those structures are connected in the relatively thick cell or how the structures function.

A new type of microscope, which takes advantage of basic science discoveries about various types of laser light, has recently been developed. It is called a confocal laser scanning microscope, and it combines several types of gas lasers to excite fluorescent dyes used to stain structures with a thick slice of tissue. The laser system scans through the tissue and sends images to a computer, which reconstructs them into three-dimensional photographs. With light photography and electron microscopy, samples have to be sliced so thin that it is not possible to follow structures such as neurons in brain tissue. The confocal laser scanning microscope allows the scientist to follow nerves to see where they attach, and also to do experiments that indicate how they function.

Another field that has advanced very rapidly in the past decade is neuroradiology — taking pictures of the brain and the rest of the nervous system. Neurologists previously relied on X- rays or gamma rays to create images of the head, spine, and extremities. X-rays reveal bones very well, but they do not show much detail in soft tissue, such as the brain or nerves.

This changed when CT (computed tomography) devices were developed about twenty years ago, using computer technology to combine and enhance many X-ray images. MRI (magnetic resonance imaging) devices were developed about ten years ago. They use magnetic energy to create images and are the preferred method of diagnosing tumors and other abnormal structures in the nervous system and other soft tissues. Experimental MRI machines can study the behavior of individual chemicals in specific parts of the brain.

While X-ray, CT, and MRI devices show structures, two new types of devices have been developed to show what is happening within those structures. PET (positron emission tomography) and SPECT (single photon emission computed tomography) reveal different intensities of chemical reactions within structures. This enables scientists to compare normal scans to those of a person with epilepsy to see, for example, if there are any differences in the way the person's brain is functioning.

One area of epilepsy research that has benefited greatly from more powerful microscopes and other scientific equipment is the study of how neurons exchange messages. This exchange occurs at a gap between neurons called the synapse. A certain electrochemical mixture must be present for the synapse to function efficiently. When a person has epilepsy, this system of neuron communication sometimes becomes overloaded. Millions of neurons get out of control and begin exchanging erroneous electrochemical messages that cause the person to behave in ways that are characteristic of a certain type of seizure.

Developmental researchers have used new knowledge about synapses to try to develop substances that can stabilize the exchange of electrochemical messages. Some of this work can be done with isolated neurons in laboratory cultures, but most of the research must be done in living animals that experience seizures, mostly mice and rats. A significant development in the past fifteen years has been the selective breeding of animal models for epilepsy. Scientists have been able to breed types of mice and rats that have seizures when given a certain chemical or other stimulus. By breeding these animals, scientists have made available thousands of animal models that can be used to test chemical compounds designed to block epileptic seizures.

The development of animal models for diseases has been accelerated and improved greatly through the current international effort to identify all the genes on the twenty-three human chromosomes. This "human genome program" has already made it possible to isolate the genetic abnormalities that result in several diseases. The genetic abnormalities have been introduced into mice, creating animal models of diseases in much less time and with much more similarity to the human form of the disease.

The availability of animal models for epilepsy now makes it possible to test thousands of compounds every year to see if they can block seizures. If a compound can block seizures in animals, other tests are done to see if the animal can function and be healthy when taking an effective dose of the seizure-preventing compound. Thanks to excellent animal models and testing procedures developed by laboratory scientists, each experimental compound can be screened in less than a week.

If a compound appears to be effective in this first phase of animal testing, it is then tested in other animals to see if it is harmful in any way. Different amounts and ways of administering the drug may also be tested. Then, after as much information as possible has been gained from animal research, the Food and Drug Administration reviews an application from the developers and decides whether to approve testing the compound in humans; this is called clinical research.

Why Is Animal Research Still Necessary?

Before discussing clinical research, it is important to understand why animal research is necessary. Throughout the history of medical research, people have wrestled with the ethics of using animals to advance human knowledge. Groups once known as antivivisectionists—today they call themselves animal rights advocates—have been active since the nineteenth century, opposing the use of animals in scientific education and research.

Animal rights advocates often claim that animal research has not resulted in any medical gains in the past. They know that most people do not receive information about the history of medicine in school or in the mass media. In fact, without animal research there would be no vaccine for polio or any other infectious disease, people with insulin-dependent diabetes would die within months because insulin would not be available, there would be no open-heart surgery or any other complicated surgical procedure, and people with epilepsy would have uncontrollable seizures because there would be no new antiepileptic medications.

Despite these advances—and many more—and the millions of people suffering the enormous toll of diseases not yet conquered, animal rights groups argue that animal research should be restricted or stopped. They assert that medical science and education should be able to proceed using cell cultures or computer simulations of biological systems. This is simply not true. Scientists are far from knowing enough about biological systems to recreate all their functioning and interacting parts in computer programs. Cell cultures do not provide functioning biological systems such as neuron networks that are needed to test antiseizure compounds. Cell cultures and computers have made it necessary to use fewer animals in some types of research, but they are far from providing a suitable alternative to living animals.

Another argument made by animal rights groups is that medical researchers receive funding for projects that involve torturing animals for no clear research purpose. This tactic takes advantage of the public's lack of information about the competitiveness of research grants and the very strict guidelines that must be followed. The NIH carefully reviews proposals for animal research to make sure that the research is necessary and that it is carried out with a minimum of distress to the animals.

Additionally, each university or research organization must have an animal research committee that is made up of some members of the outside community, often the local animal humane society representative. This committee approves applications and oversees animal research and education laboratories, making sure that repetitive or unnecessary research is not being done and that all possible steps are taken to prevent animals from suffering. The U.S. Department of Agriculture assists the NIH in holding surprise inspections of these facilities to make sure rules about cage sizes, cleanliness, and animal care are being strictly adhered to.

Animal rights activists and medical researchers actually share a common goal: achieving a world without animal research. However, animal rights activists want to have that world now, at the expense of the millions of people affected by diseases and disorders. Medical researchers and educators would also like to do away with the need for animals in research because they do not like to hurt or kill. However, medical researchers understand how little we actually know about living systems, and they therefore appreciate how important animals will be for a long time to come.

If Congress were to outlaw animal research, as animal rights activists continue to suggest, not only medical research but also medical education would stop. Our medical schools would graduate doctors who had never gone beyond a textbook or computer in learning living anatomy and physiology. Medical treatments would be frozen in time. Can you imagine going in for a new type of surgery that has never been tried on a living thing? Can you imagine taking a medication that has not been tested on animals and whose toxicity and long-term effects are therefore unknown? The fact is that no pharmaceutical company would market such a medication, and no medical school would graduate such a surgeon.

In other words, without animal research, we would live in a world without new medications and treatments for diseases such as heart disease, cancer, diabetes, and epilepsy.

Polls continue to show that 75–85% of the American public understands the importance of animal research and believes that it should continue. If you agree, it is important that you contact your representatives in Congress and in your state legislature, and that you support your local medical school or research institution. If you have a chance, take the time to provide some accurate information in response to the wishful thinking and misinformation spread by animal rights organizations.

Clinical Research

After animal research has shown that a compound or treatment is effective and safe when given to animals as similar to humans as possible, the FDA approves clinical studies. There are several steps involved in testing any new medicine or treatment on humans.

When the FDA approves human testing of a potential antiepileptic medication, for example, the first step is very limited testing on volunteers, healthy people who do not have epilepsy. This step involves a relatively small number of people who are monitored closely to see if the new treatment has any unexpected side effects or affects humans differently than it did animals. If this step is successful, the FDA approves the next step, which is testing on people whose seizures are not well-controlled by any other medication. This is usually interpreted to mean people who have four or more seizures per month.

There are many different procedures for testing a potential antiepileptic medication, but at this time all initial testing must be done on people who are eighteen years or older. Most initial testing is done in the hospital to allow neurologists to closely monitor the effectiveness and safety of the medication. Pharmacists and clinical nurses are also often involved in monitoring the patient's therapy and keeping blood levels of the experimental medication at desired levels.

If inpatient testing shows that the medication is safe and effective, the FDA can approve outpatient testing in people who meet the strictly defined indications of the clinical research project. For example, this might be males with epilepsy who are between eighteen and forty years old. The FDA wants to prevent problems in women who may become pregnant and in children and older people, although Congress has recently required that more clinical research involve women and members of different races. These limited clinical tests may last for two or three years. Then, depending on how effective and safe the medication is shown to be, the FDA may approve it for testing in other groups of people with epilepsy, including women and children. If all goes well in clinical testing, the FDA grants marketing rights, giving the pharmaceutical company authorization to market the medication for the purpose for which it has been proved effective and safe. Physicians can then prescribe it according to their professional judgment about whether it will help control a person's seizures. All serious side effects must be reported to the FDA to allow ongoing monitoring and reporting of the medication's safety.

The process that starts with testing a new compound in animals and sometimes results in its approval as a medication for sale to humans costs tens to hundreds of millions of dollars and usually takes anywhere from five to ten years. This seems too long for people with the disease or disorder it is intended to treat, especially if it is a fatal disease, such as AIDS. The FDA has shortened the time necessary to approve human use of AIDS drugs, and there may be similar improvements in efficiency with other medications.

There is a big difference between greater efficiency and reduced caution, however. No one wants to see new medications rushed onto the market before anyone knows how they will affect

rushed onto the market before anyone knows how they will affect certain groups of people over the many years that they will be used.

Besides testing new medications, clinical studies are also done to evaluate new medical devices. The past decade has seen dramatic advances in devices that improve the ability of neuroradiologists and neurosurgeons to diagnose disorders in the brain and to operate very selectively on those disorders without affecting other parts of the brain. New types of laser cutting devices and radiation therapy machines have also improved the selective nature of brain surgery. Robotic devices are also being used in connection with computers and video imaging of the interior of the brain to enable a surgeon to guide therapeutic devices to operate on structures that previously could not be safely reached.

How Can I Help Promote Epilepsy Research?

There are many ways to contribute to epilepsy research. The most obvious is by donating money for neuroscience or epilepsy studies at your local research institution or for clinical research at an epilepsy center. You can also write letters to or visit with your representatives in national and state governments to make sure they understand the importance of funding epilepsy research. You can combine your efforts with others by supporting the national research programs of the EFA.

If your child's seizures are not well-controlled, there may be a possibility of participating in a clinical research program. Although most drug trials require patients to be over the age of eighteen in early stages, younger children may be allowed to participate in later stages of the trial. Your first consideration should be whether you and your child's physician agree that the research project might help improve your child's epilepsy control and general well-being. If your child participates in such a study, it is important that you follow instructions exactly so that the information gained is as accurate and as helpful to your child and others as possible.

You can become an advocate for epilepsy research and help raise money to support various types of research projects. Each of us can help support medical research by helping to educate others about the reasons animal research is necessary, and about the dramatic advances that are being made toward the day when epilepsy and other disorders and diseases will be footnotes in history.

APPENDIX 1

FIRST AID FOR EPILEPSY: HOW TO HELP WHEN SOMEONE HAS A SEIZURE

What is epilepsy?

Epilepsy is a chronic disorder of the brain that causes seizures. There are many different causes of epilepsy—head injuries, brain infections, disorders occurring during fetal development, and many others. However, in about half of all people with epilepsy, a specific cause cannot be determined. About one percent of the population has epilepsy. Medications can control or reduce the number of seizures for most people with epilepsy. When medications do not control seizures completely, surgery may be recommended.

How can I tell if the person is having a seizure or some other health problem?

The major difference between seizures and other medical conditions that may resemble seizures is that seizures start very quickly and are usually over in a few minutes.

- If you don't know the person has a history of seizures, follow the guidelines outlined below.
- If you don't know the person, but someone else nearby does, and seems to know to to handle the situation capably, ask what you can do to help.
- If no one around knows the person, and the symptoms last more than a few minutes, call for help.
- If the person awakens and says "I'm OK," and seems OK, you probably don't need to call for help.
- Anyone who has a seizure for the first time should see a physician.

About MINCEP® Epilepsy Care

MINCEP is a national center for children and adults with all types of epilepsy. MINCEP's comprehensive patient care programs focus on the medical, surgical, social, and emotional needs of children and adults with epilepsy, using the most advanced medical technologies and research findings. MINCEP's goal is to achieve complete control of seizures without side-effects. For more information, ask your doctor or call 612-525-2400.

♦® is a registered mark and licensed to MINCEP® Epilepsy Care.

MINCEP® is a registered name and licensed to MINCEP® Epilepsy Care.

223

Generalized Tonic-Clonic Seizure
(Old name: "grand mal" seizure)

During the seizure

The person may fall, become stiff, and make jerking movements.

The person's complexion may become pale or bluish.

DO help the person lie down and put something soft under the head.

DO remove any eyeglasses and loosen any tight clothing.

DO clear the area of sharp or hard objects.

DO NOT force anything into the person's mouth.

DO NOT try to restrain the person. You cannot stop the seizure.

After the seizure

The person will awaken confused and disoriented.

DO turn the person to one side to allow saliva to drain from the mouth.

DO arrange for someone to stay nearby until the person is fully awake.

DO NOT offer the person any food or drink.

An ambulance usually is not necessary.

Call 911 or local police or ambulance **if** . . .

. . . the person does not start breathing within one minute after the seizure. If this happens, you should call for help and start mouth-to-mouth resuscitation.

. . . the person sustains an injury.

. . . the person has one seizure right after another.

. . . the person requests an ambulance.

Complex Partial Seizure
(Old name: "temporal lobe" or "psychomotor" seizure)

During the seizure

The person may:

- have a glassy stare.
- give no response or an inappropriate response when questioned.
- sit, stand, or walk about aimlessly.
- make lip-smacking or chewing motions.
- fidget with or remove clothes.
- appear to be drunk, drugged, or even psychotic.

DO try to remove harmful objects from the person's pathway or coax the person from them.

DO NOT try to stop or restrain the person.

DO NOT agitate the person.

DO NOT approach the person if you are alone and the person appears to be angry or aggressive. This is very unusual.

After the seizure

The person may be confused or disoriented after regaining consciousness.

DO stay with the person until he or she is fully alert.

Call 911 or local police or ambulance **if**. . .

. . . the person is aggressive toward you and you need help.

. . . the person sustains an injury.

What is a seizure?

Seizures are sudden, uncontrolled episodes of excessive electrical discharges of brain cells, causing a variety of sensory, motor, and behavioral changes. Seizures are the most common sign of epilepsy, although not all seizures are caused by epilepsy. A person who has more than one seizure on more than one occasion is said to have epilepsy. Nine percent of the population has a seizure sometime in their lives.

© 1991, Rev. 1992 MINCEP® Epilepsy Care. Reprinted with permission.

APPENDIX 2

DRIVING AND EPILEPSY

State	Seizure-Free Period	Periodic Medical Updates Required After Licensing	Doctors Required to Report Epilepsy	DMV Appeal of License Denial*
Alabama	1 year	Annually for 10 years from date of last seizure	No	Within 10 days
Alaska	6 months	At discretion of DMV	No	Within 15 days
Arizona	3 months, with exceptions	At discretion of MVD	No	Within 15 days
Arkansas	1 year	At discretion of DMV	No	Within 20 days
California	3, 6, or 12 months, with exceptions	As above	Yes	Within 10 days
Colorado	No set seizure-free period	As above	No	Yes
Connecticut	No set seizure-free period	As above	No	Yes
Delaware	No set seizure-free period	Annually	Yes	Yes

State	Seizure-Free Period	Periodic Medical Updates Required After Licensing	Doctors Required to Report Epilepsy	DMV Appeal of License Denial*
District of Columbia	1 year, with exceptions	Annually until 5 years seizure-free	No	Within 5 days
Florida	6 months, with exceptions	At discretion of Medical Advisory Board	No	Yes
Georgia	1 year. Less if only nocturnal seizures	At discretion of DMV	No	Within 15 days
Hawaii	1 year, with exceptions	At discretion of DMV	No	Yes
Idaho	1 year, 6 months with strong recommendation of doctor	Annually	No	Any time
Illinois	No set seizure-free period	At discretion of Medical Advisory Board	No	Yes
Indiana	No set seizure-free period	As above	No	Yes
Iowa	6 months. Less if seizures nocturnal	After first 6 months, then at renewal	No	Within 30 days
Kansas	6 months	Annually, until 3 years seizure-free	No	Within 30 days
Kentucky	90 days	On renewal	No	Within 20 days
Louisiana	1 year, with exceptions	At discretion of DMV	No	No
Maine	6 months or longer	As above	No	Yes
Maryland	90 days	As above	No	Within 15 days
Massachusetts	6 months	At discretion of Medical Advisory Board	No	Within 14 days
Michigan	6 months. Less at	At discretion of Medical	No	Within 14 days

State	Seizure-Free Period	Periodic Medical Updates Required After Licensing	Doctors Required to Report Epilepsy	DMV Appeal of License Denial*
	discretion of department	Advisory Board		
Minnesota	6 months, with exceptions	Every 6 months until 1 year seizure-free; then annually for 4 yrs.; then every 4 yrs.	No	Yes
Mississippi	1 year	At discretion of Medical Advisory Board	No	No
Missouri	6 months, with doctor's recommendation	At license renewal	No	No
Montana	6 months	No	No	Yes
Nebraska	3 months	No	No	Yes
Nevada	3 months, with exceptions	Annually	Yes	Within 30 days
New Hampshire	1 year, less at discretion of department	No	No	Within 30 days
New Jersey	1 year, less with recommendation of Neurobiological Disorder Committee	Every 6 months for 2 years, thereafter annually	Yes	Within 10 days
New Mexico	1 year	At discretion of Medical Advisory Board	No	Within 20 days
New York	1 year, with exceptions	At discretion of DMV	No	Within 30 days
North Carolina	1 year, with exceptions	Annually, less at discretion of DMV	No	Within 10 days
North Dakota	1 year. Restricted licenses available after 6 months	Annually for at least 5 years	No	Within 10 days

State	Seizure-Free Period	Periodic Medical Updates Required After Licensing	Doctors Required to Report Epilepsy	DMV Appeal of License Denial*
Ohio	No set seizure-free period	Every 6 months or 1 year until seizure-free 5 years	No	Within 30 days
Oklahoma	1 year, with exceptions	At discretion of Department of Public Safety	No	Yes
Oregon	6 months, with exceptions	Every 6 or 12 months until at least 2 years seizure-free	Yes	Within 20 days
Pennsylvania	6 months, with exceptions	At discretion of Medical Advisory Board	Yes	Yes
Puerto Rico	No set seizure-free period	As above	No	Within 20 days
Rhode Island	18 months; less at discretion of Department of Transportation	As above	No	Within 10 days
South Carolina	6 months	Every 6 months	No	Within 10 days
South Dakota	12 months. Less with doctor's recommendation	Every 6 months until 1 year seizure-free	No	No
Tennessee	6 months	At discretion of Medical Advisory Board	No	Within 20 days
Texas	6 months with doctor's recommendation, with exceptions	At discretion of Medical Advisory Board	No	No
Utah	3 months	Every 6 months until1 1 year seizure-free	No	Within 10 days

State	Seizure-Free Period	Periodic Medical Updates Required After Licensing	Doctors Required to Report Epilepsy	DMV Appeal of License Denial*
Vermont	24 months, or 6 months with doctor's recommendation	Every 6 months until 2 years seizure-free	No	Within 10 days
Virginia	6 months, with exceptions	At discretion of Medical Advisory Board	No	Yes
Washington	6 months	As above	No	Anytime
West Virginia	1 year, with exceptions	As above	No	Within 10 days
Wisconsin	3 months	At discretion of DMV	No	Yes
Wyoming	1 year, with exceptions	Annually, until seizure-free 2 years, thereafter upon license renewal	No	Within 20 days

This chart was developed for information purposes by the Epilepsy Foundation of America's Legal Advocacy Department and reflects data available as of August, 1994. Information is subject to change. This chart is not a substitute for legal advice. For further information, consult your state Department of Motor Vehicles.
* Time frames within which one must request an administrative review or hearing are given when known. Every state allows for appeal of license denial through the courts.
** Note: Non-driver I.D. cards are available in every state.

APPENDIX 3

OTHER USEFUL BOOKS

Gumnit, Robert J. *Living Well with Epilepsy*, 2nd edition. New York: Demos Vermande, 1996.

Gumnit, Robert J. *The Epilepsy Handbook: The Practical Management of Seizures*, 2nd edition. New York: Raven Press, 1995.

Stolman, Marc D. A Guide to Legal Rights for People with Disabilities. New York: Demos Publications, 1994.

INDEX

Preferred provider organizations, 31–33, 200
Pregnancy, 147–48
Preschool years, 115–18
Primidone (Mysoline®), 59
Psychogenic seizures, 106
Public transportation, as alternative to driving, 159–60

Rash, as side effect, 59, 60
Rebellious behavior, coping with, 131
Recreational drugs, 113, 131–32
Rectal anticonvulsant, use of in status epilepticus, 103
Referral, to another physician, 5, 44
Research, 211–22
    animal research, 217–19
    basic science research, 212–14
    clinical research, 219–21
    developmental research, 214–17
    epilepsy research, 221–22
Residential facilities, 167–70

Sedation, as side effect, 59
Seizure
    causes of, 3, 19–21
    definition of, 2, 14–15
    different kinds of, 16–18
    epileptic, 14–15
    nonepileptic, 14–15, 106
Self–esteem, 43, 94, 102, 119, 120, 122, 124, 130, 137, 140, 174, 187
    see also Self–image
Self–image, 2, 7, 9, 101, 110, 111, 120, 122, 128, 130
Sexuality, 145–46
Sexually transmitted diseases, 146–47
Side effects, of antiepileptic medications, 58–61
    causes of, 60
    dental hygiene and, 63–64
Simple partial seizures, 17, 57, 104
Single photon emission computed tomography (SPECT), 215
Sleep, 152
Smoking, antiepileptic medication and, 113
Social services, 209–10